100 Questions & Answers About Cancer and Fertility

Kutluk H. Oktay, MD
Cornell University Weill Medical College

Lindsay Nohr Beck
Fertile Hope

Joyce Dillon Reinecke, JD
Fertile Hope

JONES AND BARTLETT PUBLISHERS
Sudbury, Massachusetts
BOSTON   TORONTO   LONDON   SINGAPORE

World Headquarters

Jones and Bartlett Publishers
40 Tall Pine Drive
Sudbury, MA 01776
978-443-5000
info@jbpub.com
www.jbpub.com

Jones and Bartlett Publishers
Canada
6339 Ormindale Way
Mississauga, Ontario L5V 1J2
CANADA

Jones and Bartlett Publishers
International
Barb House, Barb Mews
London W6 7PA
UK

Jones and Bartlett's books and products are available through most bookstores and online booksellers. To contact Jones and Bartlett Publishers directly, call 800-832-0034, fax 978-443-8000, or visit our website, www.jbpub.com.

Substantial discounts on bulk quantities of Jones and Bartlett's publications are available to corporations, professional associations, and other qualified organizations. For details and specific discount information, contact the special sales department at Jones and Bartlett via the above contact information or send an email to specialsales@jbpub.com.

The authors, editor, and publisher have made every effort to provide accurate information. However, they are not responsible for errors, omissions, or for any outcomes related to the use of the contents of this book and take no responsibility for the use of the products and procedures described. Treatments and side effects described in this book may not be applicable to all people; likewise, some people may require a dose or experience a side effect that is not described herein. Drugs and medical devices are discussed that may have limited availability controlled by the Food and Drug Administration (FDA) for use only in a research study or clinical trial. Research, clinical practice, and government regulations often change the accepted standard in this field. When consideration is being given to use of any drug in the clinical setting, the health care provider or reader is responsible for determining FDA status of the drug, reading the package insert, and reviewing prescribing information for the most up-to-date recommendations on dose, precautions, and contraindications, and determining the appropriate usage for the product. This is especially important in the case of drugs that are new or seldom used.

Production Credits
Executive Publisher: Christopher Davis
Associate Editor: Kathy Richardson
Production Director: Amy Rose
Production Assistant: Mike Boblitt
Manufacturing Buyer: Therese Connell
Associate Marketing Manager: Rebecca Wasley

Cover Design: Jon Ayotte
Composition: Appingo
Cover Image: © Michelle Walker Photography
Printing and Binding: Malloy, Inc.
Cover Printing: Malloy, Inc.

Library of Congress Cataloging-in-Publication Data
Oktay, Kutluk H.
   100 questions and answers about cancer and fertility / Kutluk H. Oktay, Lindsay Nohr Beck, and Joyce Dillon Reinecke.
      p. cm.
   Includes bibliographical references and index.
   ISBN-13: 978-0-7637-4049-8
   ISBN-10: 0-7637-4049-7
   1. Fertility--Complications. 2. Fertility--Miscellanea. 3. Fertility, Human--Miscellanea. 4. Cancer--Complications. 5. Cancer--Miscellanea. 6. Self-care, Health. I. Beck, Lindsay Nohr. II. Reinecke, Joyce Dillon. III. Title. IV. Title: One hundred questions and answers about cancer and fertility.
   RC889.O38 2008
   616.99'406--dc22
                                        2007009993
6048

Printed in the United States of America
11 10 09 08 07   10 9 8 7 6 5 4 3 2 1

"I am a cancer survivor—but I am also a Dad. When I look at my three beautiful children and realize that they would not be here if I wasn't told to bank my sperm, I feel overwhelmed with gratitude. They are my life—they are my legacy. Every cancer survivor deserves the chance to be a parent, and this book can make it happen!"

—Lance Armstrong
Chairman
Lance Armstrong Foundation

"At first glance, cancer and infertility don't seem to have much in common. But don't tell that to a young cancer patient who dreams of one day starting a family. [These authors] cut through the science, the medical jargon, and the confusion of this medical cross-section and give us an insightful primer that will be a mainstay for patients and their doctors."

—Nancy L. Snyderman, MD
Chief Medical Editor NBC News
Associate Professor of Otolaryngology
University of Pennsylvania

"A rising issue worldwide is fertility in the patient with cancer. This is due to the fortunate coupling of increasing cancer survival in young patients and new reproductive technologies that can be applied. This book by the expert in the field covers all aspects in a thorough yet comprehensive manner. The author portrays a proper perspective, and this book is filled with gems of important information. The book is so packed with excellent information that both professionals and patients will benefit. The use of patient scenarios is extremely effective."

—Alan H. DeCherney, MD
Editor-in-Chief, Fertility and Sterility

"With nearly 700,000 cancer survivors in the United States who are younger than 40, this book is about more than fertility. It is vital . . . not only to the current and next survivors, and to those around the world, but to the professionals and caregivers, many of whom struggle finding the answers that are contained within."

—*Archie Bleyer, MD*
Adolescent and Young Adult Cancer Specialist
St. Charles Medical Center

"Lindsay Nohr Beck knows the struggles of infertility after cancer firsthand. She and her colleagues have written a meticulously researched, practical guide for everyone of reproductive age diagnosed with cancer. I wish it had existed when I was diagnosed."

—*Dan Shapiro, PhD*
Director, Medical Humanities Program
Associate Professor of Clinical Psychiatry
University of Arizona College of Medicine
Author, Mom's Marijuana: Life, Love, and Beating the Odds

"This book provides authoritative answers to the many thousands of younger people diagnosed with cancer before they have had a chance to complete their families. . . . Now current information for both men and women can be found in one place, with the perspectives both of an expert healthcare professional and from survivors who have been through the experience themselves."

—*Leslie R. Schover, PhD*
Professor of Behavioral Science
UT MD Anderson Cancer Center

"At some point, most young adults diagnosed with cancer realize that life goes on, and many will live long, fulfilling, and perhaps challenging lives after cancer. Questions about "what next"—job, career, relationships, family, children—eventually replace concerns about cancer treatment. Survivors have hundreds of questions, and this new guidebook will assist by providing some solid answers."

—Brad Zebrack, PhD, MSW, MPH
Assistant Professor
USC School of Social Work

"Cancer-related infertility is an extremely complicated, emotional, and often misunderstood subject. . . . This guide will be an invaluable resource to both males and females newly diagnosed with cancer."

—Marcia Leonard, RN, NP
Fertility Counseling and Gamete Cryopreservation Program
University of Michigan Comprehensive Cancer Center

CONTENTS

SECTION I   MEN—RISKS AND OPTIONS   1

Part 1: The Basics   3

Questions 1–5 give background information about cancer and fertility for men.

* What is infertility in men?
* Is infertility the same as impotence?
* How do cancer and its treatments affect fertility?

Part 2: Your Options Before Cancer Treatments Start   9

Questions 6–14 discuss methods for preserving your fertility.

* What is sperm banking?
* How much does sperm banking cost?
* How much sperm is enough, and how many samples should I bank?

Part 3: Your Options After Cancer Treatments End   15

Questions 15–23 address parenthood options for those who are fertile and those who are sterile after cancer treatment is over.

* After treatment, how do I know whether I am fertile?
* Will fertility ever return? If so, how long will it take?
* Is it safe for me to try to conceive naturally? Is my sperm damaged?

Part 4: Special Concerns for the Parents of Prepubescent Boys   23

Questions 24–27 explain fertility concerns unique to boys who have not yet entered puberty.

* How will my son's reproductive system be affected by his cancer treatments?
* Are there fertility preservation options for prepubescent boys?
* What should I look for as he develops?

I am dedicating this book to the "young survivor"—whether single or a couple, child, or an adult or whether the parent of a child with cancer—those who courageously deal with one of the most stressful experiences in life so that they or their loved ones can fulfill their dream of raising a family.

—Kutluk H. Oktay, MD

I would like to dedicate this book to my daughter, Paisley Jane, who was growing and kicking inside my belly as we wrote. I also dedicate it to my husband, family, friends, and physicians who made my parenthood dreams come true.

—Lindsay Nohr Beck

I dedicate this book to my doctors, who saved my life; to my father, sister, and friends who were at my bedside; and to my mother who was not only my advocate, but also fought to protect the lives that give mine purpose and weight today. I also owe a special debt to our surrogate, Yvette, who taught me the meaning of generosity; to my husband, John, whose support on this journey has been unwavering; and to Alexandra and Olivia, who define survival for me every day.

—Joyce Dillon Reinecke, JD

Life is what happens to you when you are busy planning it. Cancer happens. Nobody plans on having it, although some of us are more fortunate than the others not to experience it. When it happens, we face the utmost feeling of losing control over our body. There are countless visits to doctors' offices, many invasive tests, sometimes surgery, and finally, chemotherapy or radiation treatment. Chemotherapy and radiotherapy, although intending to attack the cancer cells, are not yet perfectly refined treatment modalities. As a result, many healthy cells in our body are targeted, and even when we survive cancer, we are destined to live with their long-term consequences.

Fertility is one of the aspects of our health that can be altered by cancer treatments. Having been a subspecialist in reproductive endocrinology and infertility, it has always been my passion to help couples achieve their biggest accomplishment in life: to raise a healthy child. These couples are otherwise healthy people who are suffering from a disability that prevents them from experiencing one of the most rewarding parts of life: childbearing. Just like cancer, infertility is also associated with the distress of losing control over your body. Having cancer and facing infertility simultaneously is a doubly daunting experience, and the stress that it creates on young people and couples is immense. As many of my patients have told me, it is sometimes more upsetting to find out that you might not have a child than being told that you have cancer.

We are fortunate to live in this century, as it brings us the modern technologic advances that enable us to deal with complex diseases such as cancer in a more effective way. Advanced cancer treatments result in high success and survival rates in many cancer types. As a result, our new task is not just to enable survival, but also to allow the survivor to live a full and healthy life. This is, in fact, a current policy recommendation by the President's Cancer Panel, which I was fortunate enough to participate in. Fertility is one of the most important aspects of quality of life, and it should be every physician's goal to help fulfill their patients' dream of having children after cancer.

Within the past 10 years, the advent of technology brought us the possibility of preserving fertility by various means that include sperm, oocyte, embryo, and ovarian tissue freezing. There are also exciting developments in the area of chemoprevention and germ stem cell technology. This book is intended to help young people with cancer cope with issues regarding cancer treatment-related infertility. Our aim is to provide information in a simplified fashion so that cancer patients and survivors can make informed decisions about whether to undergo treatment to preserve their fertility and whether and how to conceive after cancer treatment. Because this textbook is not intended to be comprehensive, it is possible that we might not have included every possible question. Instead, we included many useful online links to fill in the gaps. Of course, Lindsay, Joyce, and I are dedicated to answering your questions personally.

—Kutluk H. Oktay, MD

THIS IS WHY I WANTED TO SURVIVE

As I write this, I am a proud new mom and my perspective on cancer-related infertility has changed—intensified. As you will see from my story as it unfolds below, fertility was always important to me, but it wasn't until my husband and I heard our baby's heartbeat for the first-time that it became clear—this is why I wanted to survive!

By the age of 24, I was a two time tongue cancer survivor. My first diagnosis was at the age of 22, the day after running a marathon. I thought I was the healthiest I had ever been. Clearly, I was wrong. I was successfully treated with aggressive radiation and given a clean bill of health. However, a year and a half later, the cancer returned, this time spreading to my lymph nodes.

Armed with the wisdom from the first experience—I knew I could get through the grueling short-term side effects of cancer treatments—I was much more concerned with long-term effects. I wanted to know what I would have to deal with forever. I was less focused on issues that were temporary like hair loss and nausea, and more concerned about issues that were permanent and would affect the rest of my life, like infertility.

I was treated at California Pacific Medical Center in San Francisco, by wonderful and dedicated surgeons, Dr. Nancy Snyderman and Dr. Daniel Hartman. Of all of the doctors I saw and all of the opinions I received, they were the only two who really embraced quality of life issues—the most prominent being eating and speaking! As a result, they gave me the confidence to think about survival and make decisions upfront that would impact my future.

Thanks to their brilliance, the surgery to remove 1/3 of my tongue was a success—the cancer was gone and I could eat and speak normally. To my surprise, though, surgery had to be followed-up with an exhausting three months of chemotherapy and six additional weeks of radiation.

Everything changed with the prospect of chemotherapy.

I developed a laundry list of questions for my oncologist to answer—I wanted to know everything. At the end of our discussion about the chemotherapy, I still hadn't asked about fertility, but figured since he hadn't mentioned it, it wasn't an issue.

Later, though, that didn't satisfy me. I had to know for sure. I knew if I didn't ask I'd kick myself later. So, I called him and popped the question—will the chemotherapy make me infertile? His answer shocked me. Yes! Yes, there is a good chance it will make you infertile.

Obviously upset by his response, my doctor scrambled to put me at ease. He told me not to worry, the odds were in my favor; and then he started talking about Lance Armstrong. He went on and on about how Lance had some of the same drugs I was going to have and that he just had a bouncing baby boy.

I almost choked. First, I was irate that in our previous discussion he decided not to mention this. What gave him the right to pick and choose which side effects he told me about and which he didn't?! And, if he was hiding this, what else was he hiding?!

Then I remembered an article I just read in *his* waiting room about Lance, and became furious. That month a fashion magazine had printed an article noting how grateful Lance was that he had the foresight to bank his sperm. He was infertile.

I didn't know what to do. I was beside myself. For me, the thought of being sterile was more devastating than the cancer diagnosis itself.

Naively, until then I had never thought my situation as a matter of life and death. I beat cancer before and was confident I would again. That all changed, however, when I called Dr. Snyderman and told her I refused to have chemo in the name of fertility. She kindly, but frankly, told me that she wanted me alive in five years to think about a family instead of dead because I didn't undergo treatment.

The choice was stark—life or motherhood? The answer was obvious, but infertility was still unacceptable for me. I hated the idea of being a 24 year old, single, infertile cancer survivor. I thought that there had to be something I could do. After all, men could bank their sperm. There had to be an equivalent for women, right?

Wrong. There isn't, but there are options and I went on a quest to find them. I wasn't particularly well connected in the medical world, didn't have luxury of extra time or energy and had no idea where to start, but I refused to give up!

As a single, young woman, embryo freezing was not an option for me. I did not have a partner and the idea of donor sperm was overwhelming for me at the time. I wanted to freeze my eggs.

Through sheer persistence, dedication and fear, I proceeded to question my healthcare team, call fertility clinics, scour the Internet and reach out to cancer organizations and infertility organizations, but I came up empty handed. Even worse, everything I heard was discouraging and misleading, if not outright incorrect. I was told over and over again—"you don't have time, fertility drugs cause cancer, egg freezing is not possible" and so on.

There were several organizations addressing infertility and many addressing cancer, but where the two overlapped, there was nothing. Absolutely nothing. No one could provide me information about my situation—becoming infertile *because* of my cancer treatments.

Then, I was watching the movie *You've Got Mail*. There is a part where Tom Hanks is spending the day with his little brother and sister. His crazy "step-mom" drops off the kids and says she is off to "harvest her eggs." Now, I figured, if it was in the movie, it had to be possible, and I had to find it!

So, with renewed hope, I started repeatedly calling fertility clinics in my area. After several calls to Stanford Medical Center, I was eventually told that they had an egg freezing program, but that it was only for young cancer patients.

I was thrilled! For the first time in my life, I was happy to be the "young cancer patient."

Time was of the essence. I had to start chemotherapy in two weeks and egg freezing would take approximately 12–14 days. I saw Dr. Lynn Westphal and she was everything I needed at the time; calm, wise, patient, experienced, and ready to act quickly. She was willing to help me actively plan for the life I wanted to live and so, to me, she represented tangible hope.

I was immediately examined, advised of the costs, risks and procedural details and sent home with a bag of medicine. As a part of this process, it was clearly outlined for me that embryo freezing is more successful than egg freezing. At the time, the average success rates of egg freezing were 1–3% per egg, and Stanford had not yet had any babies born through the technique. To me, however, 1–3% was better than the alternative (sterile 0%!). And, I believe in the advancement of science. I knew that by the time I went back to use my eggs the success rates would be higher.

So, I moved forward. Despite all the appointments, medications, needles, and side effects, I relished anything that had to do with harvesting my eggs. After two weeks of self-administered shots, intense side effects and an outpatient surgical procedure, I had 29 eggs safely stored for future use. That knowledge allowed me to undergo chemotherapy and radiation as scheduled with a new sense of pride, resolve, and excitement for the future. It was the first positive in a long list of negatives. I now had a reason to fight, a reason to live.

Three months later I was cured and relieved to have my eggs waiting in the wings as a vehicle to live the life I'd always imagined.

Looking back, I know that I was extremely lucky. First and foremost, I learned my risks before starting treatment. And second, despite the fact that information was almost impossible to find, the treatments were intense and insurance didn't pay for them, I was able to preserve what was sacred to me—my fertility.

I jumped back into the real world with a vengeance.

Professionally, I felt the need to create something positive out of my experience. I started Fertile Hope—a national, nonprofit organization dedicated to providing reproductive information, support, and hope to cancer patients whose medical treatments present the risk of infertility. I was haunted by the "obligation of the cured" and hated to think that my peers were being sterilized without their knowledge, especially when so many great parenthood options existed.

Personally, I found dating the first year after cancer wasn't easy. I was rejected for my cancer history and the possibility that I might not be able to have kids one day. It was a sobering lesson for me—who knows what I would have done if I found myself in their shoes. Luckily, after kissing a number of toads, I finally found my Prince Charming, Jordan Beck.

He was everything I'd dreamt of and more. To him, cancer was part of me, but it didn't define me. We dated for a couple of years, got engaged and were excited about spending our lives together. I wanted to be a pregnant bride, but he wasn't crazy about the idea, so we decided we would start trying as soon as we were married. In the meantime, we both had our fertility tested.

Jordan's sperm count was normal. And, surprisingly, I wasn't in menopause yet. As is the case with many cancer survivors, my ovaries were damaged by the chemo that I had, so I will go into menopause early. But, I wasn't there yet. We got clearance to start trying on our own.

During this time a lot of people asked me if I regretted freezing my eggs. Absolutely, not! No one knows if menopause will hit before I finish building my family, so I am thrilled to have them there, just in case. If I never need them, great, they've given me tremendous peace of mind over the years. If I do, I'll be grateful that they are there.

We began trying right after our wedding. It was an exciting time. After several months, however, we experienced several early miscarriages. I was devastated. Why wasn't this working? Had chemo damaged my eggs genetically? Would I ever have a baby?

We immediately sought the advice of a reproductive endocrinologist, Dr. Zev Rosenwaks, the Director of the Center for Reproductive Medicine and Infertility. I was scared to death to become his patient. His reputation was bigger than life. Not to mention, I had worked with him professionally and I was mortified to think of the examination. Moreover, I wasn't in a good mental state—this felt a hundred times harder for me than cancer. I was on an emotional rollercoaster.

Dr. Rosenwaks's wisdom, confidence, and impeccable bedside manner immediately put me at ease. I relinquished control (or as much control as I am capable of relinquishing) and let him lead the way. Once again, I found myself in the presence of tangible hope.

I have come to find comfort in medicine. The problem solving had begun and, I believed, solutions had to follow.

The solutions didn't come as quickly as I would have liked, but they came. Patience is not my strong suit and having to move as slowly as my menstrual cycle was torture for me. Fortunately, Dr. Rosenwaks identified the problem—and it had a solution. Jordan had a genetic abnormality called a balanced translocation. It wasn't my eggs after all.

We were told that we could use a test called pre-implantations genetic diagnosis (PGD) in conjunction with in vitro fertilization (IVF) to test our embryos for the abnormality. Those that didn't have the defect could be transferred into my uterus to try to achieve pregnancy.

I was thrilled. Jordan was heartbroken. He felt a huge sense of responsibility and guilt. Jordan wasn't used to medical adversity. He was hung up on the problem; I was focused on the solution. Eventually, we got to the same place and, excitedly, we moved forward with IVF and PGD.

It worked!

On June 1, 2006 our healthy baby girl, Paisley Jane, was born. So, although we didn't become parents the old fashioned way or the way I anticipated we would—with my frozen eggs—we did become parents. We've been blissfully exhausted ever since. I find deep comfort knowing that no matter what happens to me—cancer or otherwise—I will live on through Paisley. She is my legacy.

—*Lindsay Nohr Beck*

Although cancer is often perceived as a disease of old age, there are thousands and thousands of young people, including children and people in their 20s, 30s, and 40s, who are diagnosed with the disease each year in the United States. In fact, every year, about 140,000 people under the age of 45 years are diagnosed with cancer. For these young patients, cancer can deal a devastating double blow. Not only are they facing the prospect of their own mortality, but many will be left infertile. The diagnosis of cancer is not just a threat to life but also to the vision of the life—a vision that typically includes a family.

Fortunately, options are available to help and to provide hope for the future. First, cancer survival rates are higher than in the past and are continuing to increase. Many young patients face very good odds of beating their disease. Second, more options are now available to help preserve fertility and become a parent after treatment is finished. New reproductive technologies are being developed and refined that may be able to help individuals who have been diagnosed with cancer to build the family they always imagined. Wherever patients are on the treatment continuum, there are many ways for them to become a parent.

Because of breakthroughs in cancer and reproductive treatments, it is becoming increasingly important that the oncology community start to address the long-term side effects of cancer treatments, such as infertility caused by chemotherapy, radiation, and/or surgery. As Americans continue to put off childbearing, more and more patients find themselves diagnosed before they have completed their families.

If you have been diagnosed with cancer and having children has always been part of your life's vision, do not let those around you minimize the value of your desire. Fighting for your ability to be a parent does not mean that you are not grateful for your own health and well-being. In fact, it means that you are hopeful about the future and that you expect to live your life as fully as you would have before you survived cancer. Therefore, you should take the time to express your desires to your oncology team.

You are not alone. Many cancer survivors have taken steps to realize this vital part of their lives and have become parents. Your oncology team should be able to explain your risks for infertility and your fertility preservation options as well as provide referrals to help you build your family when you are ready.

In the end, saving a life is more than just saving the body. It is also about preserving your dreams and your legacy, which are so often embodied in our children.

—Joyce Dillon Reinecke, JD

SECTION I

MEN

RISKS AND OPTIONS

PART ONE

The Basics

What is infertility in men?

Is infertility the same as impotence?

How do cancer and its treatments affect fertility?

More . . .

Infertility

The inability to conceive after one year of unprotected intercourse or the inability to carry a pregnancy to term.

Sperm

A man's reproductive cells, also called gametes.

Ejaculate

The fluid emitted from a man's penis during orgasm that contains sperm.

Motility

The ability of sperm to move and progress forward through the reproductive tract and fertilize the egg.

Morphology

The physical structure of organisms, including sperm.

Fertility

The ability to reproduce—in humans, the ability to bear children.

Azoospermic

The absence of sperm.

Understand that treating cancer is going to be the most important thing for a certain period of time, but there may come a day when you are in recovery and might then be glad that you [planned for] a child.

—Lisa, Wife of Esophageal Cancer Survivor

1. What is infertility in men?

For men, **infertility** is the inability to father a child. It can be further defined as the inability to conceive after 1 year of unprotected intercourse. In general, infertility occurs when you stop producing **sperm** or when your sperm is too damaged.

The World Health Organization has developed criteria to measure the normal quantity, speed, and shape of sperm. Anything below these numbers is considered low or compromised:

- Sperm concentration (quantity)—more than 20 million sperm per milliliter of **ejaculate**
- Sperm **motility** (speed)—more than 50% moving sperm in ejaculate
- Sperm **morphology** (shape)—more than 30% of sperm in ejaculate have normal shape

The average man has 60 to 80 million sperm per milliliter of ejaculate. Low or compromised **fertility** is defined as sperm concentrations of less than 20 million per cc of ejaculate, whereas sterility is generally defined as a complete absence of sperm (**azoospermic**). Some couples with slightly abnormal values may still be able to achieve pregnancy naturally or by using fertility treatments.

2. Is infertility the same as impotence?

Infertility is not the same as **impotence**. Infertility does not involve sexual functioning.

3. How do cancer and its treatments affect fertility?

Not all cancers and cancer treatments cause infertility, but some do; thus, it is important to understand your individual risks. Cancer itself can cause infertility in men. For example, some men with testicular cancer and Hodgkin's disease have low sperm counts before treatment starts. This could be due to the stress of cancer or the direct effects of the tumor.

Cancer treatments can also cause infertility. In general, the higher the dose and the longer the treatment, the higher the chance for reproductive problems. The following factors can influence your risk:

- Age
- Type and dose of medications
- Location and dose of radiation
- Surgical area
- Pre-treatment fertility status of patient

Chemotherapy, radiation, and surgery can all affect your reproductive system. **Table 1** in Appendix A shows whether your cancer treatments might put you at risk for infertility.

Chemotherapy

Chemotherapy kills rapidly dividing cells throughout the body—cancer cells and healthy cells, including sperm. Your age, the type of chemotherapy, and the dose of the medications can influence your risk. Certain chemotherapy agents are more damaging than others. Generally, **alkylating agents** are the worst.

Radiation

Radiation also kills rapidly dividing cells in or around its target area. For example, radiation to or near your **testicles** can cause infertility, but radiation to your chest will not. Radiation to your **pituitary gland** or hormone-producing areas

---

Impotence

The inability to have an erection of the penis adequate for sexual intercourse. This is also called erectile dysfunction. Being impotent does not me there is no sperm.

Alkylating agents

A family of anticancer drugs that interferes with the cell's DNA and inhibits cancer cell growth. This category of chemotherapy medications generally has the worst impact on the reproductive system. Alkylating agents include busulfan, carmustine, carzelesin, cyclophosphamide (also called Cytoxan), ifosfamide, lomustine, melphalan, porfiromycin, and semustine.

Testicles

A man's sex glands located in the scrotum, which produce sperm and testosterone.

Pituitary gland

A small gland at the base of the brain that secretes hormones and regulates and controls other hormone-secreting glands and many body processes, including growth and reproduction.

The Basics

5

Reproductive system

Organs and tissues involved in the production and maturation of gametes and in their subsequent development as offspring. In men, this includes the prostate, testes, and penis.

Bone marrow transplant

Procedure in which a patient's bone marrow is replaced with new bone marrow either from the patient (autologous) or from a matched donor (allogenic).

Stem cell transplant

A procedure involving the infusion of either a patient's own stem cells or stem cells from a donor to produce new, healthy marrow. Stem cell transplantation usually refers to the collection of the stem cells from the blood stream; collection from the bone marrow is referred to as a bone marrow transplant.

of your brain may cause infertility by interfering with normal hormone production. The location and dose of radiation will influence your risk.

Surgery

Surgery that removes all or part of the **reproductive system**, such as one or both of your testicles, may cause infertility. Accordingly, the location and scope of surgery influences your risk.

Bone Marrow and Stem Cell Transplants

Bone marrow transplants and **stem cell transplants** generally involve high doses of chemotherapy, which increases the risk of infertility. Sometimes full-body radiation is used, which also presents a high risk. The combination of both of these treatments creates an extremely high risk for subsequent infertility.

Gleevec (Imatinib)

Although research is limited, there seems to be no effect to men's fertility from **Gleevec**, and it appears to be safe to father a child while you are taking Gleevec.

During my exam, the doctors found numerous tumors in my lymph nodes and spleen as well as a 6-inch tumor wrapped around my heart. I was shocked to hear the news about my tumors and then completely devastated when the **oncologist** *told me that I might become* **sterile** *as a result of my cancer treatment.*

—Brian, Hodgkin's Lymphoma

4. Am I at risk?

Please refer to **Table 1** in Appendix A to better understand your risk of infertility after cancer. Research studies have not been conducted on every type of cancer and every type of treatment to evaluate reproductive outcome, and thus, it is not always possible to know your risk of infertility. If you have a more common type of cancer like non-Hodgkin's lymphoma, testicular cancer, or leukemia, there may be studies to help calculate your risks. Discuss your individual risks with your cancer doctor.

5. Is fertility important to me?

If you are at risk for infertility caused by your cancer treatments, it is important to think about the significance of parenting to you. You may want to consider whether you want to be a father one day and, if so, whether having a child genetically related to you is important. A few sample questions to ask might be as follows:

- Have I always wanted children?
- Would I prefer adoption to other parenthood options?
- Does it matter to me whether my children are biologically related to me?
- Am I open to using donor sperm or donor embryos?
- How many children do I want to have?
- How does my partner/spouse feel about all of these issues?

Understanding how you feel about parenthood will help you decide whether options such as **sperm banking** are worthwhile for you. For example, if you would like to have a biological child with your partner, sperm banking may be the best way for you to preserve that dream; however, if you have always wanted to adopt a child or to be a foster parent, then you might decide not to bank your sperm. It is important for you to think these decisions through because they may affect your parenting options for the rest of your life.

Gleevec (Imatinib)

Drug used to treat chronic myelogenous leukemia, gastrointestinal stromal tumors, and a number of other malignancies.

Oncologist

A doctor who specializes in the treatment of cancer.

Sterile

Unable to produce children.

Sperm banking

Freezing sperm for use in the future. This procedure can allow men to father children after loss of fertility.

It is important for you to think these decisions through because they may affect your parenting options for the rest of your life.

The Basics

PART TWO

Your Options Before Cancer Treatments Start

What is sperm banking?

How much does sperm banking cost?

How much sperm is enough, and how many samples should I bank?

More . . .

6. What is sperm banking?

Sperm banking is a simple, proven way to preserve fertility. Thousands of men have been able to bank sperm before cancer treatments and then successfully use it to have children.

Across the country, there are many sperm banks including some associated with major hospitals and/or cancer centers, where you can make an appointment to bank your sperm. If there is not a sperm bank in your area, there is also an option to order a sperm banking-by-mail kit that allows you to bank your sperm at home or in the hospital and mail it to the bank.

At the sperm bank, you will be escorted to a private room to produce a specimen that will be analyzed, frozen, and stored for future use. Some men have found it distracting or embarrassing to have family or friends with them. You are not alone if you feel this way. Do what feels comfortable to you: Go by yourself, or invite someone who you know will not make an already stressful situation worse.

It used to be recommended that you wait 2 to 3 days between each donation; however, new research shows that the quality and quantity of sperm are the same every 24 hours. Thus, you can bank sperm every day. Cancer can make some people too weak to be able to do this. Do what is feasible for you; just know that you should not make more than one deposit per day, either at the bank or through sexual intercourse. Therefore, on the days that you are making a deposit for sperm banking, you must abstain from sexual activity. After you provide the sperm sample, it is frozen and can be stored for many years until you are ready to use it. For more information about how long sperm can be frozen, please see Question 11.

The success rate of sperm banking depends on several variables. First, approximately 50% of the sperm collected will survive the freezing and thawing processes. From there, the success rate depends on the quality of your sperm, your partner's age and fertility status, and the method of assisted reproduction you use for pregnancy later. For more information about using banked sperm, please see Question 21.

7. How much does sperm banking cost?

The average national cost of sperm banking is $1,500, which includes three deposits and the first 5 years of storage. The cost can vary greatly from center to center and by geographic location; thus, it is important to compare prices in your area. Storage fees range from $350 to $600 per year. Discounts on long-term storage are usually offered if you prepay more than 1 year in advance. Some insurance companies may cover sperm banking, but it is rare, especially for the long-term storage fees. Check with your insurance company to understand what is covered under your plan.

8. How much sperm is enough, and how many samples should I bank?

There is not a definitive answer to this question. Generally, the more you bank the better. You may want to consider how many children you would like to have in the future as well as the quality of your sperm at the time you bank it. For example, if you only want one child and have very high-quality sperm, you may only want to bank one or two samples; however, if you want many children or if your sperm quality is low, you may want to bank several times.

For two weeks straight . . . I went to try to bank sperm to no avail. [I was not producing sperm.] The very last day before the transplant, I had sperm and banked two vials.

—Patrick, Acute Myelogenous Leukemia

9. What if my sperm count is low? Should I still bank?

Generally, the more sperm you have and the better the quality of the sperm, the higher your chances of achieving pregnancy.

Generally, the more sperm you have and the better the quality of the sperm, the higher your chances of achieving pregnancy. Even if your sperm count is very low or poor quality, it is possible to bank it and successfully achieve pregnancy later.

11

Sperm count

A basic assessment of sperm function, primarily involving counting the number of sperm, assessing their motility and progression, and evaluating their overall structure and form.

Intracytoplasmic sperm injection (ICSI)

A process in which one sperm is injected into an egg to facilitate fertilization.

Embryo

A fertilized egg from conception through the eighth week of pregnancy.

Embryologist

A scientist who studies the growth and development of the embryo.

Fertilization

The penetration of the egg by the sperm and fusion of genetic materials, which results in the development of an embryo.

Even if your **sperm count** is very low or poor quality, it is possible to bank it and successfully achieve pregnancy later. In the past, millions of sperm were required to make banking sperm worthwhile. Today, however, as a result of new reproductive technologies, even a single sperm may be enough to achieve pregnancy. A specific technique called **intracytoplasmic sperm injection** (ICSI) allows for the placement of an individual sperm directly into a woman's egg to create an **embryo**. For more information about ICSI, please see Question 10.

10. What is intracytoplasmic sperm injection (ICSI)?

ICSI is a procedure in which one sperm is injected into a woman's egg to create an embryo. Before the invention of ICSI, many sperm would be put together with one egg in a Petri dish in the laboratory. The goal was to have one of the sperm penetrate the egg, fertilize it, and create an embryo (which is what happens inside the woman's body when pregnancy occurs naturally). If the sperm quality was poor or there were not enough sperm, this did not always happen. With ICSI, the **embryologist** can choose the best sperm (usually the best shaped and fastest moving) and inject it into the egg with a needle. The result is a higher **fertilization** rate and, therefore, a higher pregnancy rate. ICSI has revolutionized reproductive medicine and helps thousands of men who would otherwise be infertile achieve pregnancy.

11. How long can sperm be frozen?

Sperm can be frozen indefinitely. Damage to the sperm occurs during the freezing and thawing processes—not while it is frozen. As long as sperm is successfully frozen and kept under proper conditions, it can remain frozen for many years. In 2004, a baby was born with sperm that had been frozen for 28 years, which is thought to be the oldest frozen sperm used to create a baby.

12. Is it safe to bank sperm if I have already started cancer treatments?

This is a very difficult question to answer and a very difficult decision for you to make. Although undergoing surgery has no effect on sperm or sperm production, research shows that sperm cells and the **stem cells** that create sperm can be genetically damaged by chemotherapy and radiation. DNA integrity may be compromised even after a single treatment. As a result, it is strongly recommended that you bank your sperm before starting chemotherapy and radiation.

13. What can I do if I have no sperm in my semen to bank before cancer treatment?

Some men have no sperm in their ejaculate even before undergoing cancer treatments. This may be do to your cancer or underlying infertility. Either way, you can consider freezing sperm using an advance technique called **testicular sperm extraction (TESE).**

TESE is possible for men who do not have mature sperm present in their **semen**, either before or after cancer treatments. Tissue from your testicles is **biopsied** and examined for sperm cells. If sperm cells are found, they are removed and used immediately or frozen for future use with ICSI to achieve pregnancy.

TESE is an outpatient surgical procedure. The cost of TESE ranges from $6,000 to $16,000 and is occasionally covered by insurance when performed in conjunction with other treatments. There is a wide range in costs because many variables are included: hospital fees, anesthesia, staff time, and equipment. If TESE is something that you are doing after cancer treatment along with **in vitro fertilization (IVF)**, additional costs will apply.

Stem cells

Undifferentiated, immature cells that develop into specialized cells.

Testicular sperm extraction (TESE)

A procedure for obtaining sperm by removing a small piece of testicular tissue through a small cut in the scrotum or by retrieving sperm directly from the testes.

Semen

The fluid that is released through the penis during orgasm containing sperm, seminal fluid, and glandular secretions.

Biopsy

Removal of a sample of tissue from the body for microscopic examination and diagnosis.

In vitro fertilization (IVF)

A method of assisted reproduction that involves combining an egg with sperm in a laboratory dish. If the egg is fertilized and cell division begins, the resulting embryo is transferred into the woman's uterus.

Your Options Before Cancer Treatments Start

13

After cancer, this is a great technique to consider if your **semen analysis** shows that you no longer have sperm. Studies have found viable sperm in the testicular tissue of men who have no sperm in their ejaculate after cancer treatment. One study found viable sperm in 45% of the men tested who had no sperm present in their ejaculate.

Success rates vary from center to center; thus, it is important to choose a physician or clinic with experience performing this procedure.

14. Are there other ways to protect my fertility during treatment?

If you are going to have radiation, you may want to ask about **radiation shielding**, a procedure in which a doctor places special shields around one or both of your testicles. If you are having radiation to one of your testicles or to your pelvic area, this will help to reduce the risk of damage to your fertility. There may be scatter radiation that reaches your testicles, but shielding significantly reduces the amount of radiation to the tissue. Radiation shielding does not protect from chemotherapy.

Semen analysis

The microscopic examination of semen to determine the number of sperm (sperm count), their shapes (morphology), and their ability to move (motility).

Radiation shielding

The use of a substance to block or absorb radiation so that tissues behind the shield are protected. Radiation shielding can be used to protect the reproductive system.

PART THREE

Your Options After Cancer Treatments End

After treatment, how do I know whether I am fertile?

Will fertility ever return? If so, how long will it take?

Is it safe for me to try to conceive naturally?
Is my sperm damaged?

More . . .

Assisted reproductive technologies (ART)

A term that applies to several high-tech treatments to mix sperm and eggs, including the most common, in vitro fertilization.

I knew that I'd be a parent one way or another. It was not my main focus at the time because my cancer was very rare and very aggressive, requiring me to be treated with very aggressive chemotherapy after a very invasive surgery. It wasn't until my girlfriend and I decided to be married, some 3 years later, that we returned to the issue of fertility.

—Anonymous, Malignant Mediastinal Germ Cell Tumor

15. After treatment, how do I know whether I am fertile?

Intrauterine insemination (IUI)

Process by which semen is collected and processed in a laboratory and then inserted directly into the woman's cervix or uterus to try to achieve pregnancy. This is also called artificial insemination.

After cancer treatments, you can have your fertility tested by having your sperm analyzed. At a sperm bank or urology office, you can produce a sperm sample that will be tested for quantity and quality. The results of the test will give you a better idea of what your parenthood options are. For example, if your sperm count is normal, you can try to conceive naturally. If your sperm analysis is less than ideal, you can explore **assisted reproductive technologies** such as **intrauterine insemination** (IUI)(sometimes called artificial insemination) or in vitro fertilization (IVF). Testicular sperm extraction (TESE), **donor sperm** and **adoption** are options if no sperm is present. Generally, you should wait 6 months to 1 year after cancer treatments end to do a sperm analysis because it may take that long for new sperm production to begin.

Donor sperm

Sperm from a man who is not a woman's partner for the purpose of producing pregnancy.

16. Will fertility ever return? If so, how long will it take?

Adoption

Process that creates a legal parent–child relationship between persons not related by blood.

For some men, fertility returns. For some men, it does not. As discussed above in Questions 3 and 4, your risk of infertility depends on several factors. For men who regain sperm production, it usually occurs within the first few years following treatment. If you continue to have no sperm in your ejaculate four to five years post-treatment, it is extremely unlikely that it will return.

17. Is it safe for me to try to conceive naturally? Is my sperm damaged?

Many cancer survivors are able to get pregnant naturally after cancer. If you do not experience infertility after treatment, natural **conception** may be an option.

It is important to know that your reproductive ability can be damaged in ways that may affect your ability to conceive naturally. In the short term, sperm exposed to chemotherapy or radiation may suffer genetic damage. Because it takes approximately 90 days for sperm to mature, the sperm that were developing in your body while you were undergoing your treatments may be genetically damaged. After you finish treatment and those sperm leave your body, new sperm that your body produces will not have been exposed to the chemotherapy and/or radiation that you had. Long-term damage to sperm production can occur when the stem cells that create sperm are damaged or destroyed by cancer treatments. If this occurs, you will experience permanent infertility, because without the stem cells, new sperm cannot be produced.

18. If I have frozen sperm, should I use what is frozen or try to conceive naturally?

Generally, reproductive doctors will say that "fresh is better than frozen." Semen quality decreases during the freezing and thawing process; thus, using sperm that you are currently producing is better than using sperm that was frozen. Accordingly, if your oncologist approves, you can try to achieve pregnancy naturally rather than use your frozen sperm. If you are not successful after 6 months to 1 year, you should see a reproductive specialist and re-examine the best way to move forward.

Many cancer survivors are able to get pregnant naturally after cancer.

Conception

Fertilization of a woman's egg by a man's sperm.

Your Options After Cancer Treatments End

19. How long after treatment should I wait to try to get my partner pregnant?

This is a very common question that often gets two conflicting answers. Both answers are correct, and you need to consider both as you decide how long to wait. First, most oncologists recommend waiting 2 to 5 years. Most cancers recur during this time, and thus, the doctors want to make sure that you are healthy before allowing you to try to achieve pregnancy with your partner. Everyone's medical situations are different—some survivors have to wait longer, whereas others are approved for pregnancy much earlier.

Second, from a reproductive standpoint, it is usually safe to start trying 6 months to 1 year after treatment. As explained in Question 17, this time will give any sperm that was damaged in the short term from your cancer treatments the chance to exit your system.

This question highlights the need for your cancer and reproductive doctors to work together to best determine what timeframe is safe for you, from both perspectives.

20. If my sperm analysis is good, can I let my frozen sperm go and stop paying for storage?

If sperm production returns after you have completed cancer treatment, it means that your body's ability to produce sperm has survived. If the quantity and quality of the sperm you are producing after cancer treatments are good, you may consider discarding your frozen sperm. Some men choose to keep their frozen sperm in case of a recurrence and additional resulting treatments.

21. If I have frozen sperm, how do I use it?

If you banked sperm before your cancer treatments, it can be used in one of the following two ways to achieve pregnancy later. It is important that you discuss the costs, risks, and ben-

If sperm production returns after you have completed cancer treatment, it means that your body's ability to produce sperm has survived.

Some men choose to keep their frozen sperm in case of a recurrence and additional resulting treatments.

efits of these options with your **reproductive endocrinologist** in order to decide which method should be used.

Intrauterine Insemination (IUI)

Intrauterine insemination is a procedure in which a doctor places semen inside a woman's cervix or uterus near the time of **ovulation** (when an egg drops). Sometimes this is done when she ovulates naturally, without the use of any fertility medications; however, the pregnancy rate of IUI can be significantly improved if the woman takes fertility medications to help mature one or more eggs. On average, IUI costs $300 to $700 per cycle (not including any medications), and the success rates can range anywhere from 5% to 25% per cycle. As with all reproductive techniques, success rates are based on the woman's age and fertility status, the quality of the sperm, and the experience of the reproductive center.

In Vitro Fertilization (IVF)

IVF is a technique in which a woman's eggs are removed and then fertilized with sperm in the laboratory to create embryos.

Before your partner's eggs can be retrieved, they have to be matured using injectable hormones (self-administered shots). This takes approximately 2 to 4 weeks, during which time she has regular blood tests and vaginal **ultrasounds** to monitor her progress. The process causes her ovaries to mature more eggs than they would in a natural menstrual cycle. For example, during a normal cycle, one or two eggs mature, whereas with **ovarian stimulation**, as many as 10, 20, or 30 eggs mature.

The eggs are retrieved through a 10- to 20-minute surgical procedure under general anesthesia. This is done vaginally, by **needle aspiration**. There are no scars. After the eggs are collected, they can be fertilized in one of two ways. The first method involves mixing the sperm and eggs together and allowing the sperm to find and penetrate the eggs on their

Reproductive endocrinologist

A gynecologist who has received board certification in reproductive endocrinology and infertility, following additional fellowship training in the causes, evaluation, and treatment of infertility.

Ovulation

The release of a mature egg from its follicle in the ovary. This usually occurs on approximately day 14 of a normal 28-day menstrual cycle.

Ultrasound

Procedure in which high-energy sound waves are bounced off internal tissues or organs and make echoes. The echo patterns are shown on the screen of an ultrasound machine, forming a picture of body tissues called a sonogram.

Ovarian stimulation

The administration of hormones or fertility medications to mature several eggs in the ovaries.

Your Options After Cancer Treatments End

Needle aspiration

The use of a thin, hollow needle and syringe to remove body fluid for examination.

Embryo transfer

The process of placing embryos that have been created and grown in the laboratory into the uterus to achieve pregnancy. More than one embryo can be transferred at a time, and thus, the pregnancy rate per transfer is different than the pregnancy rate per embryo or per egg.

Your partner's fertility status also plays a role in deciding which option to choose.

own. The second is to use ICSI, where individual sperm can be injected directly into individual eggs.

The resulting embryos usually grow and develop in the laboratory for 3 to 5 days. Then they can be frozen for future use or used immediately to try to achieve pregnancy. If used immediately, the embryos will be implanted into your partner's uterus during an outpatient procedure that takes less than an hour.

On average, IVF costs $8,000 per cycle, not including medications, which can range from $2,500 to $5,000.

The average success rates—live babies—per **embryo transfer** from fresh embryos are 10.6% to 36.6% in the United States. Success is based on several factors. For comparison purposes, the success rates of natural conception between a fertile man and woman are 20% to 25%.

Your partner's fertility status also plays a role in deciding which option to choose. For example, if your partner is in her 20s and appears to be in good reproductive health and your sperm quality is high, your physician may recommend using IUI. Alternatively, if your partner is in her late 30s or older or your sperm quality is moderate to poor, your physician may recommend IVF, with or without ICSI.

Here is a rough guideline on which option to choose based on how much sperm you have frozen:

- IUI—5 million motile sperm per egg per cycle
- IVF—50,000 to 100,000 motile sperm per egg per cycle
- IVF with ICSI —one sperm per egg per cycle

Although IUI is significantly cheaper than IVF, it is important to use this method judiciously so that you do not use all of your frozen sperm on the first or second cycle without ever achieving pregnancy.

22. If I do not have frozen sperm, what are my options now?

If you are infertile after your cancer treatments are complete and you do not have any sperm frozen, you can still consider fatherhood through a variety of methods:

- Testicular sperm extraction (Question 13)
- Donor sperm (Question 23)
- Adoption (Questions 81–84)

Please reference the questions listed previously here for more information about these options.

23. What is donor sperm?

Donor sperm is when you use another man's sperm to conceive a child. Donor sperm can come from an anonymous donor or from a known donor such as a relative or a friend. If you want an anonymous donor, you can select a donor from a sperm bank according to physical traits, ethnicity, or other personal characteristics that might be important to you. Reputable sperm banks screen donors based on their family background, genetic diseases, and the current health of the donor.

There are many positive aspects of **donor insemination**. First, it is one of the least expensive ways to conceive, other than natural conception. Second, your wife or partner has the opportunity to experience pregnancy and pass her genes along to the child. Third, if you carry a genetic trait that could affect the health of your child, using donor sperm avoids this risk.

The negative aspects of using donor sperm are more emotional and psychological than physical. You and your partner may mourn the loss of the ability to pass on your genetic lineage. There may be fear about your capacity to love a child that may

If you are infertile after your cancer treatments are complete and you do not have any sperm frozen, you can still consider fatherhood through a variety of methods.

Donor insemination

Artificial insemination using donor sperm.

Your Options After Cancer Treatments End

be different from you. Some religions also reject donor sperm as an option to treat infertility.

Mental health professionals in this field recommend that you take your time deciding on donor insemination, come to terms with infertility, grieve the loss of the ability to pass on your genes, and weigh donor sperm versus other options like adoption. Studies have shown that most couples who choose this option are very happy and comfortable with their choice and go on to create loving relationships with their children.

The average cost of purchasing donor sperm can range from $3,000 to $5,000. The cost of using the sperm to achieve pregnancy is additional and depends on the treatments your female partner will undergo. Donor sperm is most frequently used with an IUI cycle. If there are no fertility problems with your female partner, conception usually happens within four to six IUI cycles. The average cost of IUI is $300 to $700 per cycle (not including any medications). If IVF is needed, the average cost is $8,000 per cycle, not including medications, which can range from $2,500 to $5,000.

PART FOUR

Special Concerns for the Parents of Prepubescent Boys

How will my son's reproductive system be affected by his cancer treatments?

Are there fertility preservation options for prepubescent boys?

What should I look for as he develops?

More . . .

24. How will my son's reproductive system be affected by his cancer treatments?

As discussed in Question 3, chemotherapy, radiation, and surgery can affect the reproductive system. The dose and type of chemotherapy, and the amount and location of radiation, and the location and scope of surgery that he receives will influence his level of risk. It is important to ask his doctor about his specific risks, both short and long term. Please refer to **Table 1** in Appendix A to better understand your son's risk of infertility after cancer.

25. Are there fertility preservation options for **prepubescent** boys?

Prepubescent

At an age before puberty.

Boys who have not gone through puberty do not have mature sperm in their testicles, and thus, they cannot bank sperm.

Testicular tissue freezing

A surgical procedure to remove testicular tissue from the testes and freeze it for future use.

Boys who have not gone through puberty do not have mature sperm in their testicles, and thus, they cannot bank sperm. Currently, two techniques may offer some protection for prepubescent boys: **testicular tissue freezing** and testicular shielding.

Testicular Tissue Freezing

Testicular tissue freezing is an outpatient surgical procedure that can be done before cancer treatments start. Pieces of testicular tissue are removed and frozen for future use. This technology shows promise for the future, but is still considered experimental. There have not been any human pregnancies to date from frozen testicular tissue. The procedure is only offered at a handful of facilities across the country, and thus, it is important that you choose a doctor who has experience with this technique.

Testicular Tissue Shielding

Testicular tissue shielding may also be an option if your son is undergoing radiation to his pelvic area. External metal shields can be placed over his pelvic region to help protect the testicles from damage. Scatter radiation may cause some damage, but the shields will help decrease the overall dose of radiation to his testicles and therefore reduce damage to his fertility. This type of shield does not provide any protection from the reproductive damage caused by chemotherapy.

26. What should I look for as he develops?

After your son's treatments, there may be cancer-related effects on the growth and development of his reproductive system. In boys, puberty normally begins between 13 and 15 years old. Radiation to your son's testicles or the hormone-producing areas of the brain, such as the pituitary gland, may affect his development. Radiation to these areas may interfere with the production of **testosterone**, which can put your son at risk for either early or delayed puberty.

Early puberty can be caused by too much testosterone, which can lead to rapid bone growth and testicular enlargement before the age of 9 years. These conditions can be treated with medications.

Production of too little testosterone can cause puberty to start much later than normal or not at all. Delayed puberty can be treated with **hormone replacement therapy** (HRT), which will help your son enter puberty and maintain masculine development.

Watch your son for signs of puberty, such as facial hair, body hair, and voice changes. If you notice they are happening too early or too late, report this to his doctor.

27. When he is ready, what will his parenthood options be?

Your son's parenthood options will vary based on the effects of the cancer treatments to his reproductive system. A doctor can perform a semen analysis any time after puberty. The results of the test will help your son decide what parenthood options are right for him. Please refer to **Table 2** in Appendix A for an overview of parenthood options for men. For example, if

After your son's treatments, there may be cancer-related effects on the growth and development of his reproductive system.

Testosterone

A hormone that promotes the development and maintenance of men's sex characteristics.

Hormone replacement therapy (HRT)

The use of synthetic hormones to treat hormone deficiencies. The most common HRT involves estrogen replacement for menopausal women, but testosterone for men can also be used.

Special Concerns for the Parents of Prepubescent Boys

the results are normal, he may be able to conceive naturally. If the results show that he is producing sperm but the quality or quantity is low, he may be able to use assisted reproductive technologies. If he does not have any sperm present in his semen, options such as testicular sperm extraction, donor sperm, or adoption may all be options for him to consider.

It is important to know that sperm production can start months or years after treatment. Studies are available that document young male cancer survivors testing their fertility through unprotected sex and impregnating their partners. Until your son is ready to become a father, he should use contraceptives to avoid pregnancy, even if he believes he is infertile.

WOMEN

RISKS AND OPTIONS

PART FIVE

The Basics

How do cancer and its treatment affect fertility and menopause?

What is infertility in women?

What is premature ovarian failure (premature menopause)?

More . . .

I had a plan for where I wanted to be in life, but spending the first year of my marriage bald and infertile was not something that I'd considered! When my physician spoke to me about treatment, I got a lump in my throat, and my eyes welled with tears as I realized that the chemotherapy was about to destroy my ability to have children. It was a very empty feeling.

—Beverly, Hodgkin's Lymphoma

28. How do cancer and its treatment affect fertility and menopause?

Menopause
Stage in life when a woman stops having her monthly menstrual period. By definition, a woman is menopausal after her periods have stopped for 1 year. Menopause typically occurs in a woman's late 40s to early 50s. It is a normal part of aging, marking the end of a woman's reproductive years.

Not all cancers and cancer treatments cause infertility, but many do; thus, it is important to understand your individual risks. Cancer itself does not cause infertility in women; however, cancer treatments can cause infertility. The following factors can influence your risk:

- Age
- Type and dose of medications
- Location and dose of radiation
- Surgical area
- Pre-treatment fertility status of patient

Not all cancers and cancer treatments cause infertility, but many do; thus, it is important to understand your individual risks.

Chemotherapy, radiation, and surgery can all affect your reproductive system. In general, the greater the total doses of chemotherapy and radiation, the higher the chance is for reproductive problems.

Chemotherapy

Chemotherapy can damage or destroy your eggs. Your age, the type of chemotherapy, and the dose of the medications can influence your risk. Certain chemotherapy agents are more damaging than others. Generally, alkylating agents are the worst. Please see **Table 3** in Appendix A to see whether your chemotherapy regime has a high, medium, or low risk of infertility in women. The risk of infertility for some of the newer cancer medications is currently unknown.

Radiation

Radiation can damage your reproductive system if it is directed toward your pelvic area. For example, radiation to or near your ovaries or uterus can cause infertility, but radiation to your chest will not. Radiation to your pituitary gland or hormone-producing areas of your brain can also cause infertility by interfering with your normal hormone production. In addition, radiation to your pelvic area can cause uterine damage, which may make it difficult to maintain a pregnancy. The location and dose of radiation will influence your risk.

Surgery

Surgery that removes all or part of your reproductive system can cause infertility. Removal of one or both of your ovaries, uterus, cervix, or other reproductive organs can cause infertility. The location and scope of surgery will influence your risk.

Bone Marrow and Stem Cell Transplants

Bone marrow and stem cell transplants generally involve high doses of chemotherapy, which pose a very high risk of infertility. Sometimes full-body radiation is used in addition to chemotherapy, which further increases this risk. When whole-body radiation is used, there is also possibility of damage to your uterus. This damage can result in uterine infertility or the inability to carry a pregnancy full term.

Gleevec (Imatinib)

Although research is limited, there seems to be no effect on women's fertility from Gleevec; however, it does not appear to be safe to take Gleevec during pregnancy because of potential damage to the developing **fetus**.

When I was first diagnosed, I thought that the only thing that mattered was surviving, but as the weeks ticked by and we were still waiting for the trial to open, I started thinking that there was a possibility that someday this whole cancer thing would be behind me—or at least on the very back burner. I knew if that were the

Fetus

An unborn baby from the eighth week after fertilization until birth.

case, I would really want to have children. I also knew that my treatment might screw that up for me. I didn't want to be greedy and start thinking about kids before I even took my first dose of Gleevec, but I also didn't want to look back and regret not doing whatever I could to prevent that from happening.

—Erin, Chronic Myelogenous Leukemia

29. What is infertility in women?

Infertility is when you no longer produce mature eggs for ovulation or when you have some other condition that prevents you from getting pregnant or maintaining a pregnancy.

Infertility is when you no longer produce mature eggs for ovulation or when you have some other condition that prevents you from getting pregnant or maintaining a pregnancy. Infertility is commonly defined as the inability to conceive after 1 year of regular unprotected intercourse; however, this definition does not always apply to cancer patients. Women who have been exposed to fertility-threatening treatments should not necessarily wait 1 year. Cancer survivors are usually advised to seek counseling before trying to conceive or after 6 months of unsuccessful efforts to get pregnant.

30. What is premature ovarian failure (premature menopause)?

In addition to causing immediate infertility, cancer treatments can also cause you to go into menopause early. **Premature ovarian failure** is defined as menopause before the age of 40 years.

All women are born with a finite number of eggs—you do not grow new ones. As you age, your supply of eggs naturally diminishes until you no longer have many viable eggs, and you enter menopause. Cancer treatments such as chemotherapy, radiation, and surgery can speed up this process by damaging or destroying your eggs.

If your cancer treatments wipe out your entire **ovarian reserve,** you will be infertile and in menopause immediately after treatment. If only some of your eggs were damaged, you

Premature ovarian failure (POF)

Cessation of periods and menopause before the age of 40.

Ovarian reserve

A term used to describe the number and quality of eggs in the ovaries. Ovarian reserve decreases over time until menopause occurs and there are no more viable eggs present.

may be fertile after treatment. Even if you are fertile after treatment, your egg supply may have been reduced, and this will cause you to go into menopause earlier than you would have without cancer treatment. For example, a woman might resume **menstruation** and be fertile after receiving chemotherapy at age 25 and then go into menopause at age 35. Another woman might receive chemotherapy at age 32 and go into menopause immediately.

When I told Nick the news, he said, "I'd rather not have kids than not have you." Hearing him say that made me cry. Since I had been diagnosed, I felt a little like damaged goods, and after failing at the embryo thing, I really did. To Nick, however, I was still a catch. He had told me many times before that I was the most important thing in his life, but I also knew he really wanted to be a dad. I was telling him that may never happen, and he was completely unphased by it. "All I care about is you getting better," he said. As much I loved him for saying that, I hated to think that I—that we—might not be able to have everything we wanted in life.

—Erin, Chronic Myelogenous Leukemia

31. Does age play a role in fertility?

Age always plays a significant role in fertility for women. As discussed in Question 30, you are born with a fixed supply of eggs that diminishes as you age. When you no longer have enough viable eggs left, you are in menopause. Cancer treatments can accelerate the process by which your egg supply diminishes and, therefore, affect fertility and cause premature ovarian failure. Generally, the older you are when you enter treatment, the fewer eggs you have in your ovaries and, therefore, the more likely you are to be infertile or in premature menopause after cancer treatment.

32. Am I at risk?

Please refer to **Table 3** in Appendix A to understand better your risk of infertility and premature ovarian failure after can-

Menstruation

Periodic discharge of blood and tissue from the uterus. Until menopause, menstruation occurs approximately every 28 days when a woman is not pregnant.

The Basics

Age always plays a significant role in fertility for women.

33

cer. Research studies have not been conducted on every type of cancer and every type of treatment looking at reproductive outcome, and thus, it is not always possible to know your exact risk. If you have a more common type of cancer, such as breast cancer or leukemia, there may be studies to help calculate your risks. Discuss your individual risks with your oncologist.

When I was diagnosed with cancer, the biggest potential losses were my fertility and my hair, but unlike my hair, there was no certainty that I would regain my fertility.

—Candi, Non-Hodgkin's Lymphoma

33. Is fertility important to me?

If you are at risk for infertility from your cancer treatments, it is important to think about the significance of parenting to you. You may want to consider whether you want to be a mother one day and, if so, whether having a child genetically related to you is important. A few sample questions to ask might be as follows:

- Have I always wanted children?
- Is it important to me to experience pregnancy?
- Would I prefer adoption to other parenthood options?
- Does it matter to me whether my children are biologically related to me?
- Am I comfortable with using donor eggs or donor embryos?
- Am I open to the idea of a surrogate carrying my baby?
- How many children do I want to have?
- How does my partner/spouse feel about all of these issues?

Fertility preservation

Term used to describe procedures that protect a person's fertility. These procedures include egg and embryo freezing, sperm banking, ovarian transposition, ovarian and testicular tissue freezing, and radical trachelectomy.

Understanding how you feel about parenthood will help you decide whether **fertility preservation** options such as embryo or egg freezing are worthwhile for you. For example, if you would like to have a biological child with your partner, creating embryos might be the best way for you to preserve that dream. If you have always wanted to adopt a child or be a foster parent, then you might not choose to undergo fertility preservation. It is important for you to think these decisions through because they may affect your parenting options for the rest of your life.

I was overwhelmed by my diagnosis and had a hard time processing the consequences beyond the immediate. Since I was already in my mid 30s, I was already afraid that I would have difficulty getting pregnant, even before finding out I had cancer. So learning this only made my dream of parenthood more challenging to achieve.

—Debbie, Breast Cancer

34. Do fertility treatments cause cancer?

Years ago there were a few studies that suggested an association between the use of fertility medications and the development of certain types of cancer. Research has not shown that fertility medications cause cancer. For those with a history of certain hormone-sensitive cancers, such as breast or ovarian cancer, it is important to speak to your doctor to understand your risks. The conclusions of a few studies are noted here and may help with this discussion.

Ovarian Cancer

Although research has not shown that fertility medications cause ovarian cancer, some studies suggest that patients who are infertile may have a higher risk of getting ovarian cancer. The risk of ovarian cancer is reduced in infertile women who conceive after fertility treatments. This may mean that pregnancy helps reduce the risk.

Breast Cancer

Fertility treatments, including the associated medications, do not appear to cause breast cancer in the general population. One study, however, showed an increase in the number

It is important for you to think these decisions through because they may affect your parenting options for the rest of your life.

The Basics

Research has not shown that fertility medications cause cancer.

of women diagnosed with breast cancer within 1 year of undergoing fertility treatments. This could be because some women already had a tumor whose growth was accelerated by the treatments or because those women are being seen by doctors and are more likely to be diagnosed. There is also new evidence that people with a strong family history of breast cancer may be at higher risk of being diagnosed with breast cancer after fertility treatments, but this finding needs further confirmation.

PART SIX

Your Options Before Cancer Treatments Start

How do I decide which options are best for me?

Will I have to delay my cancer treatments
to preserve my fertility?

What is the difference between
an egg and an embryo?

More . . .

35. How do I decide which options are best for me?

Several factors will influence which type of fertility preservation method is right for you, including:

- Do you have a male partner to provide sperm?
- Are you willing to use donor sperm?
- How much time do you have before starting cancer treatment?
- Is your cancer likely to spread to your ovaries?
- What are your specific treatment risks?
- Do you have an estrogen-sensitive cancer?
- Do you have cancer in or around your reproductive system (cervix, ovaries, endometrium, etc.)?
- Do you have ethical or religious concerns about using assisted reproductive technologies?

Knowing the answers to these questions will help you select the best option for you.

If having a family is extremely important to you, do what is necessary to preserve your fertility. [Your] health is the most important piece of the equation. The two must be considered and balanced.

—Mary, Cervical Cancer

36. Will I have to delay my cancer treatments to preserve my fertility?

Fertility preservation options vary greatly, and so does the time necessary for each procedure. Egg freezing and **embryo freezing** require 2 to 4 weeks, whereas **ovarian tissue freezing** is a 1-day outpatient procedure. Some women have a 4- to 6-week hiatus between surgery and the onset of chemotherapy or radiation, which may provide a window of opportunity to preserve your fertility. If you need to start treatment immediately, you may not have time for some of the available options. If fertility preservation is something that you would

Some women have a 4- to 6-week hiatus between surgery and the onset of chemotherapy or radiation, which may provide a window of opportunity to preserve your fertility.

like to consider, talk to your oncologist about it as early as possible so that you have sufficient time before beginning your cancer treatments.

37. What is the difference between an egg and an embryo?

An egg, also called an **oocyte**, is a woman's reproductive cell. It contains only the genetic material of the woman it comes from. An embryo is an egg that has been fertilized with sperm, which means that it contains genetic material from both the woman and the man. The egg is the largest cell in a woman's body, and it contains more water than any other cell, which is what makes **cryopreservation** of eggs more difficult than embryos.

38. How long can eggs, embryos, and ovarian tissue be frozen?

Eggs, embryos, and ovarian tissue can be frozen indefinitely. Any damage that might occur happens at the time of freezing and thawing. Once frozen, they can be kept for many years. There are case reports of patients who have had embryos frozen for more than 10 years who have then gone on to achieve pregnancy.

I was 7-months pregnant when I was first diagnosed with Hodgkin's Lymphoma.

All I ever wanted in life was a big family. When the doctor told me the news [it was cancer], my first thought was for my unborn baby. The oncologist assured me it [the chemotherapy] was safe for the fetus. . . . After receiving four rounds of chemo, I was induced at 36 weeks and gave birth to a beautiful, healthy baby boy.

I was in remission for 7 months and enjoying every second of being a mother when I got the news that my cancer was back. I would need a stem cell transplant, a procedure that was almost sure to

Embryo freezing
A procedure used to cryopreserve embryos for future use.

Ovarian tissue freezing
A surgical procedure where part or all of an ovary is removed, divided into small strips and frozen for future use to try to restore hormone function and/or achieve pregnancy.

Oocyte
A cell from which an egg or ovum develops by meiosis; a woman's reproductive cell.

Cryopreservation
The process of storing biological material at low temperatures often for long periods of time.

Your Options Before Cancer Treatments Start

leave me infertile. Again, my first question was what my options were. We were told our best option was to freeze embryos, but I still didn't know if I was infertile from my first round of treatment. I found out I relapsed on a Wednesday, and by Friday, I was in the fertility specialist's office finding out whether we had any options at all. We found out that I was still fertile (yeah!) and in a perfect time in my cycle—by the next day, I was giving myself hormone shots to mass produce eggs. About a week and a half (and lots of shots) later, they extracted 16 eggs. A few days, later we had seven frozen embryos.

A year after my transplant I am cancer free. Because I took the initiative and asked the right questions, my husband and I will have the big family we always dreamed of.

—Melissa, Hodgkin's Lymphoma

39. What is embryo freezing?

Embryo freezing is the most common and successful way for a woman to preserve her fertility. It involves fertilizing your eggs with sperm in the laboratory through in vitro fertilization (IVF) and then freezing the embryos that are created. Embryo freezing requires both eggs and sperm, and thus, you need a male partner or a sperm donor.

The procedure generally takes 2 weeks from the onset of your period. On the second or third day of your period, you will start medications to mature multiple eggs in your ovaries. This requires daily, self-administered injections for approximately 10 to 12 days. You will also have frequent blood work and ovarian ultrasounds to monitor your hormone levels and the development of your eggs. You may feel bloated, uncomfortable, and moody during this time—some women compare the experience to exaggerated **premenstrual syndrome** (PMS).

When your eggs are mature, doctors will remove them in a quick outpatient surgical procedure. You will be put under a light form of anesthesia for about 10 to 20 minutes. The

---

Embryo freezing is the most common and successful way for a woman to preserve her fertility. It involves fertilizing your eggs with sperm in the laboratory through in vitro fertilization (IVF) and then freezing the embryos that are created.

Premenstrual syndrome (PMS)

Physical and psychological symptoms, including abdominal bloating, breast tenderness, headache, fatigue, irritability, anxiety, and depression, that occur in the days before the onset of menstruation and cease shortly after menses begins.

procedure is done vaginally with an aspirating needle, and thus, there are no incisions or scars from the treatment. Once removed, the eggs will be fertilized in the laboratory with sperm to create embryos. The embryos will develop in the laboratory for 3 to 5 days. The embryos that develop successfully will be frozen for future use. Not all of the embryos may develop—some may not continue to grow in the laboratory. For example, one woman might have 15 eggs extracted but only 12 embryos developing in the laboratory several days later.

When you complete your cancer treatments and are ready to think about getting pregnant, the embryos can be thawed and transferred into your uterus. From one to five embryos can be placed in your uterus at one time, depending on your age and the quality of the embryos. In general, for patients younger than 35 years, there is a trend toward limiting the maximum number of embryos transferred to two.

The success rates—live babies—per embryo transfer from frozen embryos are 19.1% to 30.6% in the United States. For comparison purposes, the success rates of natural conception between a fertile man and woman are 20% to 25%. Success rates vary based on several factors:

- Age at time of retrieval
- Quantity and quality of eggs retrieved
- Quantity and quality of embryos frozen
- Stage of embryos frozen or used
- Experience and success rate of your reproductive center

Tens of thousands of babies have been born worldwide from embryo freezing. As noted previously here, embryo freezing can take approximately 2 weeks after the onset of your period. Depending on how your menstrual cycle coincides with your cancer treatments, this may result in anywhere from 2 to 6 weeks necessary to freeze embryos.

Tens of thousands of babies have been born worldwide from embryo freezing.

40. How much does embryo freezing cost?

As reported by the American Society of Reproductive Medicine (ASRM), the average cost of in vitro fertilization is $8,000, not including medications, which can range from $2,500 to $5,000.

As reported by the American Society of Reproductive Medicine (ASRM), the average cost of in vitro fertilization is $8,000, not including medications, which can range from $2,500 to $5,000.

Though we rarely talked about it, deep down I think we both knew we wanted to marry each other someday. We just didn't want to be one of those couples that picks out their kids' names on their third date and plans their wedding before they've had their first fight. We didn't want to count our chickens before they hatched, so to speak. Sure it was fun to fantasize about our life together, and sometimes we couldn't help but picture what kind of house we would have or what type of parents we'd be. But talking about our future too much always put a strange pressure on things, so we tried to avoid it. Plus, we, and by we I mostly mean Nick, had some growing up to do. We were too young, too unsettled in our lives, especially financially. When grilled by our family and friends, we'd say, "If we're as in love and as compatible as we are now in 3 or 4 years, then we'll do it." We were big on throwing in the "if": if we're still together, if we still love each other, if we get married. But once the embryo stuff came up, we no longer had the luxury of if.

—Erin, Chronic Myelogenous Leukemia

41. What if I don't have a partner to provide sperm?

If you do not have a husband or male partner, you may want to think about using donor sperm. Donor sperm can come from either an anonymous donor or from a known donor, such as a relative or a friend. If you want an anonymous donor, you can select a donor from a sperm bank according to physical traits, ethnicity, or other personal characteristics that might be important to you. Reputable sperm banks screen donors based on their family background, genetic diseases, and the current health of the donor.

If you do not have a husband or male partner, you may want to think about using donor sperm.

I had to choose a sperm donor. It's amazing how many "choices" I had, and thanks to the Web, I had the ability to select a donor. Thanks to a tall 6'4", blue-eyed, dark-haired doctor from California who is well traveled, loves sports, and the outdoors, I selected you! (Who wouldn't with those credentials?)

—Amy, Non-Hodgkin's Lymphoma

42. What is egg freezing?

Egg freezing is an experimental fertility preservation option for women who either do not have a male partner, do not want to use donor sperm, or have ethical or spiritual objections to embryo freezing. The process for removing the eggs from your body is the same as in embryo freezing (please see Question 39 for a detailed description of the process). The key difference is that the eggs that are removed from your body are not fertilized with sperm. They are frozen as is and, therefore, contain only your genetic material.

Because eggs are large cells that contain a lot of water, they are more difficult to freeze than embryos. During the freezing process, the water inside the egg can form ice crystals, which can damage the cell and its chromosomes. There are currently two ways to freeze eggs: **slow freezing** (sometimes called controlled-rate freezing) and **vitrification** (fast freezing). The primary differences in the two methods are the techniques used in the laboratory to freeze and thaw the eggs. More than 90% of the babies born from egg freezing today involved the slow-freezing protocol, which was the technique that was developed first. The use of vitrification is increasing.

Although it is difficult to compare them side by side, it is generally accepted that egg freezing is not as successful as embryo freezing, but the technology is improving rapidly. One recent study compiling the results of all published egg-freezing data showed that the live birth rate per embryo transfer using frozen eggs is 21.6%. Comparatively, as reported by the Centers

Egg freezing is an experimental fertility preservation option for women who either do not have a partner, do not want to use donor sperm, or have ethical or spiritual objections to embryo freezing.

Egg freezing

A procedure used to extract mature unfertilized eggs from the body and store them for future use.

Slow freezing

A technique used to freeze eggs and embryos. Cooling and warming rates are controlled to reduce the risk of ice crystal formation and damage to the egg or embryo.

Your Options Before Cancer Treatments Start

Vitrification

Method of egg "freezing" that involves rapid cooling with high concentrations of cryoprotectants to reduce the formation of ice crystals.

The average pregnancy rate for a fertile couple is 20% to 25%.

Approximately 200 babies have been born worldwide from egg freezing.

for Disease Control, in 2005, in the United States the average live birth rate using fresh embryos ranged from 43.3% (under the age of 35) to 14.9% (over the age of 40) and the live birth rate from frozen embryos ranged from 31.8% (under the age of 35) to 15.6% (over the age of 40). The average pregnancy rate for a fertile couple using natural conception is 20% to 25%. The same study showed that success rates with egg freezing are on the rise, especially with the fast-freezing technique. As with embryo freezing, many factors account for the success rates of egg freezing, including the following:

• Age at time of retrieval
• Number of eggs retrieved
• Quantity and quality of embryos created later
• Experience and success rate of your reproductive center

Approximately 200 babies have been born worldwide from egg freezing.

Egg freezing can take approximately 2 weeks after the onset of your period. Depending on how your menstrual cycle coincides with your cancer treatments, this may result in anywhere from 2 to 6 weeks necessary for the process.

When my oncologist first sat down with me to discuss the risks of chemotherapy, he happened to mention the slight risk of infertility. He also said that if the cancer ever comes back or doesn't respond to chemotherapy, I would have to endure a bone marrow transplant, which would definitely cause infertility. This was the one time I cried. This news devastated me more than having the cancer itself. What was I supposed to do? I've always wanted to have a family and the experience of being a mother.

Freezing my eggs was my own "insurance policy" that allowed me to focus on surviving cancer and not on the subsequent risks that fed my mind with thoughts of depression, anger, and confusion. Most would think that having cancer would cause these destructive thoughts, but it wasn't for me. Freezing my eggs was a must—no questions asked.

—Antoinette, Hodgkin's Lymphoma

43. How much does egg freezing cost?

The average cost of egg freezing is $8,000, not including medications, which can range from $2,500 to $5,000. Some centers offer egg freezing for free or at a discounted rate if it is done as part of a research study.

Know that there are hundreds of thousands of people in your situation—you are not alone. Also, keep the faith that there are many ways to become a parent.

—Karen, Sarcoidosis

44. What is ovarian tissue freezing?

Ovarian tissue freezing is an experimental technique that may be a good option for you if you do not have sufficient time before cancer treatments, if it is not safe for you to undergo hormonal stimulation, or if you have not yet entered puberty. Doctors remove all or part of one ovary in a one-hour outpatient surgical procedure. You will be put under general anesthesia for this minimally invasive surgery, which is done with a "keyhole" incision in your belly button. No hormone stimulation is needed before the surgery. The removed ovary is divided into thin strips of tissue, which contain hormone-producing cells and immature eggs. The tissue is then frozen and stored for future use. This procedure is still experimental, and fewer than four babies have been born worldwide to date.

Ovarian tissue freezing is an experimental technique that may be a good option for you if you do not have sufficient time before cancer treatments, if it is not safe for you to undergo hormonal stimulation, or if you have not yet entered puberty.

Of all of the fertility preservation options available for women, ovarian tissue freezing requires the least amount of time—1 day for surgery. Accordingly, it can usually be squeezed into most cancer treatment timelines.

This technology shows promise for the future, but is still considered experimental. The procedure is only offered at a handful of facilities across the country, and thus, it is important that you choose a doctor who has experience with this technique.

45. How much does ovarian tissue freezing cost?

As with many fertility preservation options, the procedure is still considered experimental and may not be covered by insurance. The cost of freezing the tissue averages $4,000 to $5,000, and hospital costs for the surgery may be as much as $10,000 to $15,000.

Some centers offer ovarian tissue freezing for free or at a discount as part of a research study.

Check with your physicians as well as your health insurance plan to understand better what costs you will be responsible for. Some centers offer this procedure for free or at a discount as part of a research study.

46. What is in vitro maturation?

In vitro maturation (IVM) is an experimental procedure in which doctors retrieve immature eggs from your ovaries, instead of mature eggs, as is done with egg and embryo freezing. This means that the standard hormones used in most fertility treatments are not needed.

Once removed, the immature eggs are matured in the laboratory, instead of inside of your body. After they are matured, they can be frozen as eggs or fertilized and frozen as embryos. IVM has been effective with some groups of infertility patients, specifically those with polycystic ovarian syndrome (PCOS), but published studies with cancer patients are not yet available; thus, it is hard to know whether those successes will transfer to cancer patients. The benefits of this procedure from the perspective of a cancer patient are that it takes less time and fewer medications than egg or embryo freezing.

47. How much does IVM cost?

The cost of one round of IVM egg harvesting and freezing is approximately $5,000 dollars (Canadian). We note Canadian dollars here because the center with the most experience with this technique is the McGill Reproductive Centre in Montreal. Some centers in the United States also offer IVM, but there are no available data on average costs. Discounts may be available when it is offered as part of a research study.

48. If I do not have time or choose not to undergo fertility preservation before I start my cancer treatments, is there any way that I can lower my risk of infertility?

Several techniques can be used to try to reduce the damage to your ovaries caused by chemotherapy and/or radiation. These techniques include:

Ovarian shielding

If you are having radiation to your abdomen, your doctor can place external shields over the site of your ovaries to reduce the damage from radiation. **Ovarian shielding** does not protect the ovaries from damage from chemotherapy.

Ovarian transposition

Ovarian transposition involves surgically moving the ovaries out of the radiation field to decrease the amount of radiation they are exposed to and, therefore, the damage to your fertility. The ovaries may later be moved back to their original position. When the ovaries are moved out of the pelvic area and pinned up higher in the abdomen, the blood supply to the ovaries can be compromised. This technique only protects from radiation, not chemotherapy. In addition, ovaries may still receive radiation because of scatter in the abdomen. As a result, average success rate is approximately 50%.

Ovarian shielding

The use of external shields to protect the ovaries from radiation.

Ovarian transposition

A surgical procedure in which one or both ovaries are moved up into the abdomen so that they are out of the field of radiation.

GnRH analogues

Hormones similar to the naturally occurring gonadotropin-releasing hormone.

Ovarian suppression

Intervention to temporarily stop the functioning of the ovaries.

Follicle

A small sac in the ovary where an egg develops.

GNRHa

GNRH analogues (GnRHa) (gonadotropin-releasing hormone analogue) treatment is an experimental option for fertility protection during chemotherapy. It is a medication taken via monthly injection or, in some cases, one injection every 3 months. The medication causes the ovaries to temporarily shut down. It is believed that by shutting down the ovaries ("**ovarian suppression**") and putting the body in a temporary prepubertal state that there may be a reduction in the damage to the **follicles** where eggs develop from the chemotherapy. The medication is usually given at least a week before cancer treatment begins so that it can take effect before chemotherapy starts. Some studies have suggested that GnRHa may be a successful option; however, there is some skepticism in the medical community about its effectiveness.

There is also concern that in hormonally sensitive cancers, such as breast cancer, these drugs may alter your response to chemotherapy. Research clearly shows that GnRHa does not protect when very high doses of cancer drugs or radiation therapy is used. Because GnRHa shuts down your ovaries, it can cause side effects common in menopause, such as hot flashes and vaginal dryness. These symptoms are temporary, and GnRHa does not cause permanent menopause.

GnRHa comes in several forms manufactured by different companies. The cost varies, but can average $500 per month (per injection). It can be ordered by your oncologist, obstetrician/gynecologist, or a fertility specialist and many insurance companies cover the costs.

PART SEVEN

Your Options After Cancer Treatments End

After treatment, how do I know whether I am fertile?

If I get my period back after treatment,
does that mean that I'm fertile?

Will fertility ever return? If so, how long will it take?

More . . .

I am now the mother of 2-year-old boy/girl twins, born in 2003, almost 10 years to the day from my original diagnosis. Fortunately, I had no problems conceiving, but I realize that I am extremely lucky. It makes me angry for others who maybe weren't so lucky because they didn't get the right information or advice at the right time.

—Heidi, Ewing's Sarcoma

49. After treatment, how do I know if I am fertile?

There is no perfect fertility test, but there are ways to assess your fertility status after treatment. First, if you resume menstruation within 1 year after cancer treatment, it is a good sign; however, having your period does not guarantee fertility. Second, you can have your **follicle-stimulating hormone** (FSH) and **Estradiol** (E2) levels tested. These are measured by simple blood tests that are usually done on day 2 or day 3 of your period. This can be done by your obstetrician/gynecologist or a reproductive endocrinologist. If you are not having regular periods, this test can still be performed to determine whether you are menopausal. Third, an ultrasound of your ovaries may be helpful in assessing your ovarian reserve (the number of eggs in your ovaries).

Many cancer survivors chose to see a reproductive endocrinologist after treatment or when they are ready to start a family. Meeting with a fertility specialist before you start trying to get pregnant may give you a better idea of your fertility status and which options are right for you, which can help you avoid wasting time and money.

Generally, if you do not achieve pregnancy after 1 year of having unprotected sex around the time of ovulation, you should see a fertility specialist. If you are 35 years old or older, it is generally recommended that you see a fertility specialist after 6 months of trying to conceive. If you are a cancer survivor,

Follicle-stimulating hormone (FSH)

A hormone produced by the pituitary gland that stimulates the growth of eggs in the ovaries. This hormone is used to help gauge ovarian reserve.

Estradiol (E2)

The principal hormone produced by the growing ovarian follicle. Blood estradiol levels are used to help determine follicle growth during an in vitro fertilization cycle.

Meeting with a fertility specialist before you start trying to get pregnant may give you a better idea of your fertility status and which options are right for you, which can help you avoid wasting time and money.

your **egg reserve** may have been damaged, and thus, it is often recommended that you see an infertility specialist before trying to conceive or after only 6 months of trying.

50. If I get my period back after treatment, does that mean that I'm fertile?

Although menstruation is generally a good sign that your reproductive system is functioning, it is not the same as fertility. Many women resume menstruation after cancer and are fertile; however, others resume menstruation and are infertile. Getting your period back after cancer treatment may be an indication that you have not entered menopause yet, but fertility begins declining approximately 10 years before you stop menstruating. This means that you may have your period, but still have trouble conceiving. Moreover, some women still have irregular menstruation-like bleeding even though they have become menopausal. For more information about how to know whether you are fertile after treatment, please see Question 49.

Getting your period back after cancer treatment may be an indication that you have not entered menopause yet, but fertility begins declining approximately 10 years before you stop menstruating.

51. Will fertility ever return? If so, how long will it take?

If your period is going to return, it usually happens within 6 months to 1 year after you complete your cancer treatments, but occasionally, it can take longer than that. If your period has not returned or is very irregular more than 1 year after completion of treatment, you may want to consider fertility testing.

52. Will I remain fertile? Am I still at risk for early menopause?

For women, fertility is never permanent. Fertility declines as you age. Thus, if you are fertile after the completion of your cancer treatments, it does not mean that you will remain fertile forever. As discussed previously, cancer treatments can cause a depletion of your egg supply that can cause premature menopause and infertility. Chemotherapy or radiation might have damaged a significant portion of your egg reserve, bringing you much closer to menopause than you would otherwise be. Because there is no way to know when **ovarian failure** may happen, some women choose to freeze embryos, eggs, or ovarian tissue after treatment. This is especially relevant if you are still many years away from being ready to start or complete your family, if your oncologist will not allow you to get pregnant for many years, or if you face the potential of having more sterilizing cancer treatments such as additional chemotherapy or a bone marrow transplant in the future. In addition, if you are fertile right now but your hormone levels such as FSH and E2 are high, you may have a shorter timeframe for childbearing than you would have had under normal circumstances.

Ovarian failure

The inability of the ovary to respond to hormone stimulation, usually caused by the absence of eggs (oocytes).

53. Is it safe for me to try to conceive naturally? Are my eggs damaged?

Many women are able to get pregnant safely and naturally after cancer treatment. If you do not experience infertility or go into menopause right after treatment, natural conception may be an option for you.

Many women are able to get pregnant safely and naturally after cancer treatment.

It is important to know that the eggs in your ovaries that were exposed to radiation and/or chemotherapy can be harmed—some may be damaged, some destroyed altogether and others may remain intact. Generally, the eggs that are the most damaged are those that are in the process of maturing while they are exposed to your cancer treatments. The time required for those eggs to exit your system is approximately 6 months; therefore, from a reproductive standpoint, it is usually recommended that you wait for at least that long to try to get pregnant. Your oncologist, however, may want you to wait longer for reasons related to your own health and particular diagnosis, and thus, it is important to consult with your healthcare team before trying to achieve pregnancy.

This question highlights the need for your cancer and reproductive doctors to work together to determine what time-frame is best for you, from both perspectives.

54. If I froze eggs, embryos, or ovarian tissue before cancer treatments but am fertile after treatment, should I use what is frozen or try to conceive naturally?

From a practical standpoint, it is easiest and most cost-effective to try to conceive naturally. If that does not happen, you may want to consider fertility treatments using fresh eggs or embryos. During this time, your frozen eggs, embryos, or tissue does not age, and thus, you do not need to rush to use them.

Even though you may be fertile now, as you age you still may face the risk of premature ovarian failure. If you can conceive naturally and save your frozen eggs, embryos, or tissue in case you need them in the future, that is always recommended, especially if you want to have a large family.

55. How do I treat menopause after cancer?

If you are in premature menopause after cancer, it may be necessary for you to take hormone replacement therapy (HRT). The birth control pill provides sufficient HRT for most young adult cancer survivors, but other HRT options are also available. The benefits of HRT taken during what would normally be your reproductive years are generally considered to outweigh any risks associated with taking HRT. In extremely rare cases, women who are in premature menopause conceive naturally. Although birth control pills would prevent that, if you do not want to forfeit this possibility, there are hormone replacement protocols that do not interfere with fertility. HRT can be an important survivorship treatment, so it is important to talk to your oncologist about your options.

Even though you may be fertile now, as you age you still may face the risk of premature ovarian failure.

Additionally, it is often recommended that young women in menopause take calcium and vitamin D supplements. Bone density measurements should be done periodically, and if thinning of the bone is detected, bisphosphonate (bone thickening drugs) treatment may be recommended.

In women with history of breast or endometrial cancer, the safety of HRT is unknown; calcium, vitamin D, and bisphosphonates may be the only recommended treatments.

56. How can I become a mother now?

There are many ways to become a mother after cancer, even if you are no longer fertile. If you have frozen eggs, embryos, or ovarian tissue, you can use them. If not, you can consider adoption, **donor eggs**, **donor embryos**, or surrogacy.

Being diagnosed with breast cancer did not change my desire to become a parent, but it did make me realize that it may not be possible to become a parent or that it certainly would not be as easy as I thought to have a family. If anything, it created a greater sense of urgency because I knew that my "biological clock" was ticking, yet due to my cancer and related treatment, there would be a time when it would not be possible to start a family. Because of this combination of factors, it made me consider fertility alternatives that I had not considered at that point in my life.

—Mary, Breast Cancer

57. How do I use my frozen embryos?

When you are ready to get pregnant, you will work with a reproductive specialist who will thaw your embryos and transfer them to your uterus. You may have to take medications to build the lining of your uterus so that the embryos will **implant** and grow. Even if you are in menopause, you can still carry a baby.

In non-cancer cases, most thawed embryos are transferred into the uterus during a natural cycle, which means that no

---

There are many ways to become a mother after cancer, even if you are no longer fertile.

Donor eggs

Eggs from the ovaries of a fertile woman that are donated to an infertile woman to be used in an assisted reproductive technology procedure.

Donor embryos

Embryos donated from one couple to another person or couple.

Implantation

The process of attachment of the embryo to the endometrial lining of the uterus.

Even if you are in menopause, you can still carry a baby.

medications are required. This option is considered the easiest and is best used with women who ovulate regularly and normally. Another option is called a programmed cycle, which requires your cycle to be controlled by medications, some of which may be self-injected. This is generally used if you are older, not ovulating, or in premature ovarian failure. The programmed cycle includes multiple ultrasounds and blood work.

Frozen embryos are stored in small groups so that you do not have to thaw and use them all at the same time. For example, if you have 10 embryos frozen, you may decide to thaw three the first time you try to achieve pregnancy. You do not have to thaw and use all 10 embryos in one cycle. The number of embryos that will be put into your uterus at once depends on your age and the quality of the embryos. Generally, between three and six will be thawed, and one to five will be transferred per cycle. There is a trend toward implanting no more than two embryos at a time.

Three out of four embryos are generally expected to survive the rigors of freezing and thawing. Success rates vary from center to center, but overall embryo survival rates are higher than 50%. This is different than the pregnancy rate—embryo survival rate is how many survive freezing and thawing.

The costs of using your embryos to get pregnant will vary from center to center and will depend in part on whether you undergo a programmed cycle and what types of medications are used. There are no good available data on the average cost. But this is a great question for your reproductive specialist to answer.

58. How do I use my frozen eggs?

The process of using your frozen eggs is the same as the process of using frozen embryos, except for one key difference: The eggs need to be fertilized with sperm after they are thawed. When you are ready to try to conceive, some or all of your frozen eggs will be thawed and fertilized using your partner's or donor sperm to create embryos. Fertilization will be done using intracytoplasmic sperm injection (ICSI), which is when a single sperm is injected directly into the egg. For more information about ICSI, please see Question 10. This technique is preferred with thawed eggs because the shell of the egg hardens during the freezing process. The resulting embryos would then be transferred to your uterus just like in an IVF cycle. If you use your partner's sperm, he will have to make a sperm deposit at the laboratory on the same day, near the same time that your eggs are thawed.

This is a new area of medicine, and thus, there are no good data available on average costs. Generally, you would need to pay for the thawing process, ICSI (which averages $2,500), and the transfer (which depends greatly on the method of transfer, medications needed, and the center you use).

59. How do I use my frozen ovarian tissue?

Currently, the only way to use frozen ovarian tissue is to thaw the tissue and re-implant it into your body. This is a highly experimental procedure, but research to expand the efficacy of this technique is actively being pursued. The ovarian tissue can be reimplanted into one of three places:

• Pelvic area (its original location)
• Under the skin in forearm
• Under the skin in the abdomen

In successful transplants, the reimplanted ovarian tissue has started to produce hormones and maturing eggs again. There are two potential benefits of reimplanting tissue. First, if you are in menopause from your treatments, hormone function may be restored. To date, there have been a few cases in which hormone production has been restored for periods of up to 2 years. Second, eggs within the re-implanted tissue can be matured with injectable hormones, collected and fertilized in the lab to create embryos. Those embryos can then be used to try to achieve pregnancy.

The average cost of transplanting the tissue back into your body may range from $10,000 to $15,000. However, if the tissue is transplanted under the skin, the costs will be less as the procedure(s) is done under local anesthesia. From there, the costs of using the resulting egg(s) to try to achieve pregnancy are similar to standard IVF, which averages $8,000 per cycle, not including the medications, which can range from $2,500 to $5,000.

There is ongoing research investigating the possibility of using in vitro maturation (IVM) with ovarian tissue freezing so that one day re-implantation of the stored tissue may not be necessary. If the research is successful, in the future, it may be possible to extract immature eggs from the frozen tissue, mature the eggs in the laboratory, and then use them to try to achieve pregnancy with IVF. This technique would avoid the costs and potential complications of surgery to re-implant the tissue, including the concern of reintroducing cancer cells back into your body.

I have always wanted to become a parent. My diagnosis didn't change my desire. It just changed the way I viewed how that was going to be accomplished. I am not a parent yet, but I have hope that I will be.

—Debbie, Breast Cancer

60. What are donor eggs and embryos?

Donor eggs are eggs that are given to you by another woman. Donor embryos are donated by a couple. Donor eggs and embryos can be provided to you by either known or anonymous donors.

There are many positive aspects of donor eggs and embryos. First, even if you no longer have your own eggs, you have the opportunity to experience pregnancy. Second, if you choose donor eggs, your partner can pass his genes along to the child. Third, if you carry a genetic trait that could affect the health of your child, using donor eggs or embryos avoids this risk.

The negative aspects of using donor eggs or embryos are more emotional and psychological than physical. You and your partner may mourn the loss of the ability to pass on your genetic lineage. There may be fear about your capacity to love a child that may be different from you. Some religions also reject donor eggs or embryos as an option to treat infertility. Mental health professionals in this field recommend that you take your time in deciding on donor eggs and embryos, come to terms with infertility, grieve the loss of the ability to pass on your genes, and weigh these options versus other options like adoption. Studies have shown that most couples who choose donor options are very happy and comfortable with their choice and go on to create loving relationships with their children.

Egg donation

The process by which a fertile woman donates her eggs to be used in the treatment of others.

If you decide on an anonymous egg donor, you can find her through your fertility clinic or through an **egg donation** agency. You can choose a donor based on physical characteristics, ethnic background, educational background, or other criteria that you may value. Most donors are between 21 and 29 years old and have undergone basic psychological, medical, and genetic screening. It is important to ask how candidates are screened, as some centers do more extensive tests and background checks than others.

Donor embryos usually come from couples who have extra embryos after having undergone their own fertility treatments to have children. You can usually find donor embryos through your fertility clinic or through a donor embryo agency. As with donor eggs, you may consider the physical characteristics, ethnic background, education, and occupation of the couple donating the embryos.

Food and Drug Administration (FDA) regulations now exist that require clinics using donor eggs and embryos to perform screening for certain infectious diseases, as well as meet certain storage and reporting standards.

Food and Drug Administration (FDA) regulations now exist that require clinics using donor eggs and embryos to perform screening for certain infectious diseases, as well as meet certain storage and reporting standards. When you are working with a center, you should check that they comply with these basic FDA requirements. In addition, the American Society of Reproductive Medicine (ASRM) has guidelines concerning the screening and compensation of donors. To protect your own health and to ensure that recognized industry standards are being met, you may want to ask the clinics that you are working with whether they comply with the ASRM recommendations for egg and **embryo donation**.

Prices vary greatly from clinic to clinic, but you should expect to pay between $15,000 and $20,000 for one donor egg or embryo IVF cycle. This includes:

- Donor eggs or embryos, $5,000
- One cycle of IVF, $8,000
- Medications, $2,500 to $5,000

Using donor eggs, the average live birth rate per cycle is a 51%. This is higher than standard IVF because donors are generally younger than standard IVF patients, and they do not have fertility issues.

I met my husband at my weakest point; he was a roommate in a large beach house. He saw me after chemo and bought me a dog bed so that I wouldn't have to rest on a cold bathroom floor. We fell in love and progressed on the high-speed love program, and eloped after a few weeks. We decided to consider parenthood after I got through the worst of the illness, and after four IVF attempts, we have 2-year-old son born via a surrogate gestational carrier (my womb mate)—an astounding woman who carried our biological son for us. It is a miracle, and we are dazzled by our great fortune every day and are full of gratitude for [my womb mate] and for our miraculous son, Jack.

—Karen, Sarcoidosis

Your Options After Cancer Treatments End

Embryo donation
Please see donor embryo.

Using donor eggs, the average live birth rate per cycle is a 51%. This is higher than general IVF because donors are generally younger than standard IVF patients, and they do not have fertility issues.

PART EIGHT

Pregnancy After Cancer

How long after treatment should I wait
to try to become pregnant?

Does pregnancy after cancer cause recurrence?

If I am in menopause, can I carry a baby?

More . . .

61. How long after treatment should I wait to try to become pregnant?

This is a very common question that often gets two conflicting answers. Both answers are correct and need to be considered as you decide how long to wait.

First, most oncologists recommend waiting 2 to 5 years. Most cancers recur by this time, and thus, they want to make sure that you are healthy before allowing you to try to get pregnant. With that being said, everyone's medical situations are different—some survivors may be advised to wait for several years, whereas others are approved for pregnancy much earlier.

Second, from the reproductive standpoint, it is usually recommended that you wait a minimum of 6 months after treatment. As discussed earlier, the eggs that are the most damaged because of their exposure to chemotherapy and radiation are those that were in the process of maturing during your cancer treatments. The time required for those eggs to exit your system is approximately 6 months.

This question highlights the need for your cancer and reproductive doctors to work together to best determine what timeframe is safe for you from both perspectives.

62. Does pregnancy after cancer cause recurrence?

Research on this topic is limited, but reassuring. Current available research suggests that pregnancy after cancer does not cause recurrence, even after breast cancer.

63. If I am in menopause, can I carry a baby?

It is possible to carry a baby if you are in menopause. You will not be able to get pregnant naturally, but you can use previously frozen eggs, embryos, or ovarian tissue. You can also use donor eggs or embryos. As long as your reproductive system is otherwise healthy, you should be able to carry a pregnancy.

64. Do cancer survivors have a higher rate of miscarriage?

This is only a concern for a small percent of patients who had radiation to their pelvic area. **Miscarriage**, **preterm delivery**, and low birthweight infants are more common in women who received radiation affecting their uterus. This commonly occurs in the setting of total body radiation given before **hematopoietic stem cell transplantation** (HSCT) procedures. If this is a concern for you, a specialist can evaluate whether there is damage to your uterus. To date, research does not suggest a higher rate of miscarriage after exposure to chemotherapy or radiation to other parts of the body.

65. Are there additional health risks associated with pregnancy for cancer survivors?

There are a variety of long-term health risks associated with chemotherapy and radiation treatments, such as damage to your heart or lungs, that could complicate your ability to carry a pregnancy. Many survivors undergo tests such as **echocardiograms** to make sure their hearts are healthy. To understand your specific health risks, you should ask your oncologist about the possible side effects of your treatment before getting pregnant. If he or she feels that you are at risk for pregnancy complications, you may need to work with a high-risk **obstetrician**.

66. What if I cannot carry a pregnancy? What is surrogacy?

When a woman is unable to carry a pregnancy but would like to parent her biological child, she can turn to the help of a **surrogate**—a woman who will carry her pregnancy for her. A family member or a friend can act as a surrogate.

Pregnancy After Cancer

Miscarriage
Early pregnancy loss, usually before 20-weeks gestation. This is also called spontaneous abortion.

Preterm delivery
Birth occurring earlier than 37 weeks of gestation. This is also known as premature birth.

Hematopoietic stem cell transplant (HSCT)
A procedure involving the infusion of either a patient's own stem cells or stem cells from a donor to produce new, healthy marrow.

Echocardiogram
A noninvasive test in which sound waves are used to produce an image of the heart.

Obstetrician
A doctor who specializes in pregnancy, labor, and delivery.

Surrogate
A woman who carries a pregnancy for another person or couple.

Alternatively, you may want to find someone through an agency or a clinic that is willing to work with you.

There are two types of surrogacy:

Traditional surrogacy

This involves using your partner's sperm to inseminate the surrogate. This means that the baby that is born would be genetically related to your partner and the surrogate. Traditional surrogacy is being used less and less.

Gestational surrogacy

This arrangement occurs when a woman, usually referred to as a "gestational carrier," becomes pregnant through IVF, with an embryo that is not genetically related to her. Any embryos that are transferred to the surrogate are created by you and your partner, and therefore, the baby is genetically related to you.

If you cannot use your own eggs, donor eggs or embryos can be used. If donor eggs are used, they can be fertilized with your partner's sperm so that the child will be genetically related to him.

The hysterectomy was necessary, but in saving my life, I also destroyed such an integral part of my future. I was very depressed and hopeless about my future. Then I realized I still have my ovaries and could maybe someday have a surrogate give birth to our baby.

—Tara, Cervical Cancer

PART NINE

Unique Concerns with Breast and Gynecologic Cancers

Are there special reproductive concerns for
breast cancer patients and survivors?

How do breast cancer treatments affect fertility?

Is it safe for me to undergo
in vitro fertilization (IVF)?

More...

Being diagnosed with breast cancer at age 37 was a complete and utter shock. At first, all I could think about were the treatments, the side effects, and whether I was going to live. After I was pretty sure I was going to survive, my focus shifted to getting through treatment as painlessly as possible and, more importantly, thinking about the future, especially fertility preservation. Being one of the crowd in the waiting room at the fertility clinic became something to look forward to, and even the battle with my insurance company about paying for my embryo freezing (which I won!) was something positive. Even now, more than 4 years after diagnosis, the thought of my frozen embryo waiting to be used—or not—as the future dictates, brings me hope.

—Anne, Breast Cancer

67. Are there special reproductive concerns for breast cancer patients and survivors?

Breast cancer patients have special reproductive concerns because breast cancer can be hormone sensitive. Tumors that are hormone sensitive may grow when exposed to certain hormones. Because some fertility preservation procedures, assisted reproductive technologies, and even pregnancy will affect hormone levels in the body, they may be of concern for some breast cancer patients.

68. How do breast cancer treatments affect fertility?

Chemotherapy can increase your risk of infertility or premature ovarian failure because it reduces your egg supply. Several chemotherapy protocols that are available to treat breast cancer have an effect on fertility. Accordingly, you may want to ask your oncologist for more information about the success rates, side effects, and associated fertility risks of the different breast cancer treatment protocols.

The types of surgery and radiation generally used to treat breast cancer do not usually affect your reproductive system,

Breast cancer patients have special reproductive concerns because breast cancer can be hormone sensitive.

and thus, they rarely affect fertility. If you have surgery to remove your ovaries as part of your treatment, fertility will be affected. Please refer to Question 72 for more information.

I was 39 years old when I was diagnosed with breast cancer. I was still ovulating and had no children. The doctors never told me that after chemotherapy treatment that I would be in a premature state of menopause and my opportunity to have children gone. I kept wondering when my periods would return and finally when I asked was told never.

—Nancy, Breast Cancer

69. Is it safe for me to undergo IVF?

No one can answer this question with 100% certainty, as current research results are limited. Because breast cancer can be hormone sensitive and fertility medications increase **estrogen** levels, standard fertility treatments may be considered unsafe in women with breast cancer by some specialists. Even if your cancer is labeled estrogen receptor negative, there may still be some small number of estrogen-sensitive cancer cells in your body that, theoretically, can be fueled by high estrogen levels.

Many doctors are opposed to giving standard fertility drugs to patients with estrogen sensitive cancer, whereas some believe that, because fertility medications are only used for a short period of time, the transient effect of raising your estrogen levels is acceptable, especially if you undergo chemotherapy later. This is a very personal decision that involves evaluating your own medical situation, your desire to undergo IVF, as well as approval from your oncology team. Until further research is done to show that standard fertility treatments are safe, you may want to consider enrolling in a study that is testing alternative ways to stimulate your ovaries so that your eggs or embryos can be frozen. For more information about these alternative methods, please see Question 70.

Because breast cancer can be hormone sensitive and fertility medications increase estrogen levels, standard fertility treatments may be considered unsafe in women with breast cancer by some specialists.

Estrogen

A hormone produced in both men and women that has a variety of functions. In women, estrogen regulates the development of secondary sex characteristics, including breasts, regulating the monthly cycle of menstruation, and preparing the body for fertilization and reproduction. In breast cancer, estrogen may promote the growth of cancer cells.

70. Are there fertility treatments that limit estrogen exposure for women with breast cancer?

Most infertility treatments use hormones to mature multiple eggs in your ovaries during a menstrual cycle. This is called standard stimulation. These hormones can raise a woman's estrogen levels, a special concern for breast cancer patients. Many breast tumors are sensitive to estrogen, and higher estrogen levels may speed the growth of some cancer cells.

Hormones are not required for all infertility treatments, but they are usually needed for embryo freezing and egg freezing. There are several alternative ways to obtain mature eggs that may be safer for women with breast cancer. The methods listed here may reduce exposure to the high estrogen levels of standard stimulation, which may lower the risk that the hormones will speed up tumor cell growth.

There are several alternative ways to obtain mature eggs that may be safer for women with breast cancer.

Egg and Embryo Freezing

Below are some alternative assisted reproductive techniques that can be used with egg and embryo freezing.

Natural cycle: As the name suggests, only eggs that mature naturally during your menstrual cycle are retrieved. No extra hormones are used, but the success rates are low. Generally, only one egg develops each month. Anywhere from zero to two eggs are retrieved.

Tamoxifen

A medication that blocks the effects of estrogen on many organs, such as the breast. Tamoxifen can be used with standard fertility medications to block the effects of estrogen.

Tamoxifen* stimulation: Many women use tamoxifen in breast cancer treatment to protect the breast from the effects of estrogen. This may seem like a contradiction, but used in

---

*These drugs should never be used during pregnancy, but when they are used for fertility treatments, they are discontinued before egg collection, and thus, developing embryos are not exposed to them.

different doses, tamoxifen may also be used as an infertility treatment. Tamoxifen stimulates the ovaries, causing an average of two eggs to be collected in each cycle. The chance of getting at least one embryo is better than with a natural cycle. Tamoxifen can also be used in conjunction with standard hormones. The standard hormones help mature multiple eggs, while the tamoxifen shields the breasts from the surging hormones. Early results show that more eggs can be retrieved this way than with tamoxifen alone. Both of these methods are still investigational. Longer patient follow-up is needed to make sure that they are absolutely safe.

Aromatase Inhibitors: Aromatase inhibitors are drugs that block most of the body's estrogen production. They are usually given to postmenopausal women as adjuvant treatment. Using aromatase inhibitors with standard stimulation keeps the total estrogen level in the body lower. This reduces the risk that the hormones used for egg maturation will speed up tumor growth. With this method, doctors have obtained as many eggs as they can from standard IVF treatments, with the number of eggs dependent on the woman's age. For a woman in her mid 30s, this can average from 10 to 12 eggs per cycle. This method is still experimental; however, no increase in cancer recurrence has been noted in preliminary studies.

Aromatase inhibitors
Medications that lower the amount of estrogen in the body.

Ovarian Tissue Freezing

Ovarian tissue freezing is a procedure where doctors remove part or all of one ovary in a 1-hour outpatient surgical procedure under anesthesia—no hormone stimulation or medications are required leading up to the surgery. The ovary is divided into strips of tissue, each of which contains hormone-producing cells and immature eggs. The tissue is then frozen and stored for future use. Please see Question 44 for more information.

In Vitro Maturation

In this process, a doctor retrieves immature eggs from your ovaries, instead of mature eggs, as done with egg and embryo freezing. This means that the standard medications usually used in fertility treatments are not needed. The immature eggs are then matured in the laboratory, instead of inside you. Once matured, they can be frozen as eggs or fertilized and frozen as embryos. This method is experimental. You will have to seek centers that have expertise in this technique or that offer this method as a part of a research study. Please see Question 46 for more information.

After my cancer treatment, I went through IVF in a clinical study for breast cancer patients. The treatment used an aromatase inhibitor to maintain lower estrogen levels during the IVF cycle for breast cancer patients who are estrogen receptor positive. The frozen embryos were thawed and implanted, which resulted in the birth of our son. If it were not for the protocol and treatment, it is likely that we would have a child. When you have been diagnosed with cancer, you are concerned with anything that may increase the likelihood of recurrence. At the same time, if you have not started a family, you may have a tremendous sense of urgency because of your age. This provides an option that lets you go through IVF yet minimizes the estrogen in your body which hopefully reduces the risk of cancer recurrence.

—Mary, Breast Cancer

71. Does pregnancy after breast cancer increase my risk of recurrence?

Pregnancy after cancer does not trigger recurrence, even after breast cancer.

Research to date, although limited, is reassuring. The consensus today is that pregnancy after cancer does not trigger recurrence, even after breast cancer. More research, including prospective studies, is still needed. For example, the data on the safety of pregnancy for *BRCA* gene carriers are extremely limited. In the meantime, it is important to talk to your doctor to see whether pregnancy after breast cancer is safe for you.

Individual factors such as age, cancer stage, years since diagnosis, and treatments undergone can all affect your risk.

72. If I want to have my ovaries removed after breast cancer, how does this affect my parenthood options?

As a part of breast cancer treatments, some women decide to have their ovaries removed. This is called oophorectomy. For example, some women with very aggressive recurrent or metastatic breast cancer may have their ovaries removed to stop estrogen production in the body, and thereby reduce their risk for recurrence. Similarly, women who are positive for the BRCA mutation may, as a prophylactic measure, have their ovaries removed to lower their risk for both breast and ovarian cancer.

If you have your ovaries removed, you will be in menopause. You will not be able to get pregnant through intercourse or assisted reproductive technologies. If the rest of your reproductive system is left in place and is healthy, you would be able to carry a pregnancy even if you are in menopause. This means that you may be able to achieve pregnancy using previously frozen eggs, embryos, or ovarian tissue. Alternatively, if you are concerned about carrying a pregnancy, you could use those eggs, embryos, or tissue in conjunction with a surrogate. If you would like to carry a pregnancy but did not undergo fertility preservation before your ovaries were removed, you can use donor eggs or embryos.

73. Is it safe to get pregnant if I am taking tamoxifen?

It is not safe to get pregnant while taking tamoxifen. If you accidentally become pregnant while you are on tamoxifen, call your doctor immediately. Studies show that tamoxifen may be associated with fetal abnormalities if taken while pregnant.

It is not safe to get pregnant while taking tamoxifen.

74. Are there special reproductive concerns for gynecologic cancer patients?

There are many surgical options for gynecologic cancers that may help preserve your fertility.

The types of reproductive concerns for gynecologic cancers are similar to those for other cancers, but your risks may be higher and your options may be different because of the location of your cancer—in or around your reproductive system.

In general, gynecologic cancers are treated with surgery, chemotherapy, and/or radiation therapy. All of these treatments can be harmful to your fertility, especially because they are directed at your reproductive system. The location of surgery, your age, the type and dose of drugs used, and the location and dose of radiation can influence your risk. A gynecologic oncologist can help you understand how your treatments might affect you.

75. Are there fertility-sparing surgeries that I should consider?

There are many surgical options for gynecologic cancers that may help preserve your fertility. The options are directly related to the type of cancer you have, and thus, the following options are discussed by cancer type.

Cervical Cancer

Fertility-sparing surgery may be an option for early-stage cervical cancer. The most minimally invasive cervical cancers are stage IA1. For this early-stage cancer, a procedure called **cervical conization** may be possible. During cervical conization, a surgeon removes only the central part of the cervix. It is a relatively simple outpatient procedure that can be fertility-sparing. Many successful pregnancies have been reported after cervical conization.

If cervical cancer is limited to the cervix, but is stage IA2 or IB1, a **radical trachelectomy** may be possible. Radical trachelectomy is a major surgical procedure that is performed

Fertility-sparing surgery

General term used to describe specific types of gynecologic surgery for women with ovarian or cervical cancer.

Cervical conization

Surgery to remove a cone-shaped piece of tissue from the cervix and cervical canal. Conization may be used to diagnose or treat a cervical condition. This is also called cone biopsy.

Radical trachelectomy

A fertility-sparing surgical procedure used for women with early-stage cervical cancer. The procedure removes most of the cervix but preserves the uterus, allowing for the woman to later carry a pregnancy.

through the vagina or abdomen. Although it includes removal of most of the cervix and the tissue around the cervix, the remainder of the uterus is left in place, which means that you may be able to carry a pregnancy later. During a future pregnancy, a suture (or **cerclage**) may be used to help hold the pregnancy inside the uterus. Because most of the cervix is removed, there is a higher risk for delivering a premature baby or losing the pregnancy very early. This procedure is usually combined with removing the lymph nodes in the pelvis to make sure that the cancer did not spread to other areas. If it did spread to the lymph nodes, alternative treatment such as radiation, chemotherapy, or a **hysterectomy** may be needed.

Radical trachelectomy is one of the newest fertility-sparing procedures. It is offered only in a few centers in the United States, but an increasing number of centers will offer this option in the future. There is sufficient experience with it and enough successful pregnancies for it to be an option to consider. It has been estimated that radical trachelectomy can be offered in up to 50% of cervical cancer patients instead of traditional, more aggressive surgery.

If you have a more advanced cervical cancer that may also require radiation, ovarian transposition may be an option. Ovarian transposition is a minimally invasive surgical procedure in which the ovaries are moved out of the pelvis and pinned up in the abdomen out of the radiation field (it does not protect from chemotherapy). When the ovaries are moved out of the pelvic area and pinned up higher in the abdomen, the blood supply to the ovaries might be compromised. Ovaries may still receive radiation because of scatter in the abdomen. As a result, average success rate is approximately 50%.

Endometrial Cancer

Most cancers of the uterus are **endometrial** cancers. The standard surgical procedure for endometrial cancer is a hys-

Cerclage

A surgical procedure used to keep the cervix closed during pregnancy.

Hysterectomy

Surgery to remove the uterus and sometimes the cervix. When the uterus and part or all of the cervix are removed, it is called a total hysterectomy. When only the uterus is removed, it is called a partial hysterectomy.

Endometrium

The lining of the uterus which grows and sheds during a normal menstrual cycle and which supports a foetus if a pregnancy occurs.

terectomy, which is the surgical removal of the uterus. This is sometimes combined with the removal of both **fallopian tubes** and both ovaries (**bilateral salpingo oophorectomy**). Removal of both ovaries causes an abrupt halt in estrogen production, a condition called surgical menopause.

If you have early-stage, low-grade endometrial cancer, **progestin hormonal treatment** may be a substitute for surgery. Progestin treatment is the use of hormones that cause the endometrial cancer to regress. This treatment requires a very careful initial evaluation and close follow-up. If the cancer regresses, pregnancy can be attempted naturally or by IVF.

With this method, however, there is a risk that the cancer may return or progress. Because endometrial cancer is also estrogen sensitive, hormonal stimulation may also be risky. Aromatase inhibitors can be used to avoid estrogen exposure and to freeze eggs or embryos before additional treatments that may be necessary, such as surgery. Please see Question 76 for more information.

Ovarian Cancer

Ovarian cancer may affect one or both ovaries. If only one ovary is cancerous, depending on the tumor type, you may be able to have fertility-sparing surgery. The surgery might include removal of the cancerous ovary, but would leave the unaffected ovary and the uterus. Generally, this operation would also include biopsies to make sure that the cancer is limited to one ovary.

The ovarian cancer types that are most likely to be candidates for fertility sparing surgery are as follows:

- Borderline tumors
- Invasive epithelial ovarian cancer (stage 1A)
- Malignant ovarian germ cell tumors
- Ovarian sex cord-stromal tumors (granulosa-cell tumors and Sertoli-Leydig cell tumors)

Fallopian tubes

A pair of tubes attached to the uterus, one on each side, where sperm and egg meet in normal conception.

Bilateral salpingo oophorectomy

Surgery to remove the fallopian tubes and the ovaries.

Progestin hormonal treatment

Treatment for endometrial cancer to block estrogen, the hormone that cancer cells need to grow.

If you retain one ovary and your uterus, you may be able to get pregnant naturally later, if your doctor feels that this is a safe option for you.

76. Is the use of hormones for assisted reproduction safe for people with gynecologic cancers?

Some infertility treatments use hormones to mature multiple eggs during a menstrual cycle, which is called standard stimulation. Using standard stimulation protocols can raise a woman's hormone levels, which can be unsafe for some gynecologic cancer patients and survivors. For example, it might not be safe to use standard stimulation when endometrial or ovarian cancers are present. The following are some alternative assisted reproductive techniques that do not require standard stimulation:

Using standard stimulation protocols can raise a woman's hormone levels, which can be unsafe for some gynecologic cancer patients and survivors.

Natural Cycle IVF

As the name suggests, only eggs that mature naturally during your menstrual cycle are retrieved. No extra hormones are used, but the success rates are low. Generally, only one egg develops each month, but anywhere from zero to two eggs may be retrieved.

Aromatase Inhibitors IVF

Using aromatase inhibitors with standard stimulation keeps the total estrogen level in the body lower. This reduces the risk that the hormones will speed up tumor growth. With this method, doctors have obtained as many eggs as they can from standard in vitro fertilization (IVF) treatments, with the number of eggs dependent on the woman's age. For a woman in her mid 30s, this can average from 10 to 12 eggs per cycle. This method is still experimental; no increase in cancer recurrence has been noted in preliminary studies.

These drugs should never be used during pregnancy. When they are used for fertility treatments, they are discontinued before egg collection, and thus, developing embryos are not exposed to them. Because they have a short half-life in the body (2 days), they are generally cleared form the circulation within a week. Accordingly, they may be used during fertility treatments but not during pregnancy.

Ovarian Tissue Freezing

Ovarian tissue freezing is a procedure where doctors remove one or both ovaries in a 1-hour outpatient surgical procedure under anesthesia. No hormone stimulation or medications are required leading up to the surgery. The ovary is divided into strips of tissue, each of which contains hormone-producing cells and immature eggs. The tissue is then frozen and stored for future use. Please see Question 44 for more information.

In Vitro Maturation

In vitro maturation (IVM) is when doctors retrieve immature eggs from your ovaries, instead of mature eggs as done with egg and embryo freezing. This means that the standard medications usually used in fertility treatments are not needed. The immature eggs are then matured in the laboratory, instead of inside you. After matured, they can be frozen as eggs or fertilized and frozen as embryos. Please see Question 46 for more information.

Tamoxifen IVF

Tamoxifen is sometimes used as a fertility medication for breast cancer patients undergoing IVF; however, this is not an option for endometrial cancer patients because tamoxifem stimulates the growth of endometrial cells.

PART TEN

Special Concerns for the Parents of Prepubescent Girls

How will my daughter's reproductive
system be affected?

What should I look for as she develops?

Are there fertility preservation options
for prepubescent girls?

More . . .

I spent the first few years after treatment convincing myself that I didn't want children because I thought that the option wasn't available to me. I thought adoption wouldn't be possible for a cancer survivor, and I didn't know that there was such a thing as donor egg or that it would even be possible for me to carry a pregnancy. I also spent many years deliberately avoiding a look into the future or entertaining the crazy notion that I would be alive to have children one day. I became an expert at living for the present and denying that I might have to confront my own future and the health implications of cancer treatment at some point. I do want children, and as my outlook eventually expanded over the years, it came as a huge relief that it is a possibility after all!

—Karen, Pediatric Rhabdomyosarcoma

77. How will my daughter's reproductive system be affected?

Your daughter was born with a limited number of eggs in her ovaries. Normally, the number of eggs would decrease over time until she enters menopause around 50 years old. However, chemotherapy and radiation may destroy or damage her eggs. This can cause immediate infertility or premature ovarian failure in the future.

Your daughter may get her period at a normal age and be fertile; however, damage to her egg supply from cancer treatments may cause her to enter menopause early.

Infertility occurs when she no longer has a sufficient level of mature eggs for ovulation or has another condition that prevents her from getting pregnant or maintaining a pregnancy. Premature ovarian failure (or early menopause) is defined as the loss of fertility before 40 years old. Your daughter may get her period at a normal age and be fertile; however, damage to her egg supply from cancer treatments may cause her to enter menopause early. For example, a young woman may undergo treatment at age 16 and resume menstruation and fertility but go into menopause at age 25.

In addition, radiation to your daughter's pelvic area may cause uterine damage. This damage to her uterus may make it difficult to maintain a pregnancy.

78. What should I look for as she develops?

In girls, puberty normally begins between the ages of 9 and 15 years old. Your daughter's cancer treatments could affect her development by causing her to enter puberty early or to go into premature ovarian failure.

Early puberty can be caused by radiation to hormone-producing regions of the brain. This causes the development of breasts and other sexual traits before the age of 8 years. Medications can temporarily stop this process.

Premature ovarian failure can occur if your daughter's egg supply is damaged or destroyed by chemotherapy or radiation. If this happens, your daughter may require hormone replacement therapy (HRT) to start puberty and menstruation. The birth control pill provides HRT for most young adult cancer survivors. The benefits of HRT at your daughter's age are generally considered to outweigh the risks. Discuss the risks and benefits of HRT with your daughter's doctor to understand whether it is right for her.

Your daughter's cancer treatments could affect her development by causing her to enter puberty early or to go into premature ovarian failure.

79. Are there fertility preservation options for prepubescent girls?

If your daughter has not yet entered puberty, she cannot freeze eggs or embryos. Although it may be physically possible for her to undergo egg and/or embryo freezing cycles, there are currently no centers offering this because of both medical and ethical concerns. Currently, ovarian tissue freezing is the only fertility preservation option available before puberty and it is still experimental, but there are also some techniques that may be used to protect her ovaries during radiation treatment.

Ovarian Tissue Freezing

Although ovarian tissue freezing holds a lot of promise, it is still very experimental. Doctors can surgically remove either an entire ovary or a part of an ovary. The tissue is then frozen and stored for future use. Years later, the tissue can be thawed and reimplanted. In successful transplants, the tissue starts producing hormones and maturing eggs. This would be a benefit if your daughter goes into early menopause. This procedure is only offered at a handful of facilities across the country, so it is important that you choose a doctor who has experience with this technique.

Ovarian Shielding

If your daughter is receiving radiation treatment to the abdominal area, her doctor can place external shields over the site of her ovaries to protect them from the effects of the radiation. Ovarian shielding does not protect against chemotherapy.

Ovarian Transposition

This involves surgically moving the ovaries out of the radiation field and pinning them back until radiation treatment is completed. When the ovaries are moved out of the pelvic area and pinned up higher in the abdomen, the blood supply to the ovaries might be compromised. Ovaries may still receive radiation because of scatter in the abdomen. As a result, average success rate is approximately 50%. The ovaries may later be moved back to their original position. Alternatively, eggs can be collected through your abdominal skin for in vitro fertilization treatment. If you daughter is postpuberty, the full range of fertility preservation options is available to her. Ovarian transposition does not protect against chemotherapy.

There are several ways for your daughter to become a parent after cancer.

80. When she is ready to think about parenthood, what will her options be?

There are several ways for your daughter to become a parent after cancer. Many successful options exist for cancer survivors who want to have children. Please refer to **Table 4** in Appendix A for an overview of parenthood options for women. When your daughter is ready to be a mother, it is possible that there will be even more choices available.

If your daughter is fertile after treatment, she may be able to get pregnant through natural conception or through assisted reproductive technologies, such as IVF. If she is fertile but worried about going into menopause before she completes building her family, she may want to consider fertility preservation options, such as egg or embryo freezing after she completes her cancer treatments.

If your daughter is infertile or is unable to carry a pregnancy, she may consider options such as donor eggs or embryos, surrogacy, or adoption.

Most doctors agree that pregnancy after cancer is safe for pediatric survivors and will not increase your daughter's risk of recurrence. It is important to talk to your daughter's doctor to understand whether and when pregnancy is safe for her.

Most doctors agree that pregnancy after cancer is safe for pediatric survivors and will not increase your daughter's risk of recurrence.

Finally, depending on the cancer treatments that she underwent, she may have additional concerns. Some types of chemotherapy can cause undetected damage to her heart or lungs, which can be exacerbated by the added physical stress of pregnancy. In addition, if your daughter received pelvic radiation, her uterus may have suffered some damage that could cause complications such as miscarriage or premature birth. Tests can be done to check for this type of damage, but they are not always conclusive. In general, women treated for childhood cancer should consult a high-risk obstetrician before trying to get pregnant.

OTHER CONSIDERATIONS

PART ELEVEN

Adoption

What types of adoption are there?

Is it possible to adopt if you have a history of cancer?

What are the average costs of adoption?

More . . .

81. What types of adoption are there?

Adoption is an excellent option for anyone wanting to become a parent. There are many different types of adoption:

Independent Adoption

Independent adoption is when the birth parent(s) place the child with the adoptive parent(s) without using an agency. The parties may find each other through family, friends, or the Internet. Independent adoption is not legal in all states. Where it is legal, it is advisable (and sometimes required) to have an attourney involved with the process, which can happen very quickly. This may be an inexpensive option relative to other adoption options.

Agency Adoption

A private agency adoption is when an adoption agency works as an intermediary between the birth parent(s) and the adoptive parent(s). Agencies generally charge fees for the services and have waiting lists of adoptive parents who have been screened and approved. In addition, agencies may either be general or sometimes specialized in certain types of adoptions, such as placing children of certain ethnicities.

Public Agency Adoption

Public agency adoption is when the state provides adoption services for children in state custody. Most of these children are in foster care until their birth parents rights are terminated and they are matched with an adoptive family. There is little or no cost, and in contrast to private agency adoption, there is usually a waiting list of children. Sometimes financial assistance is provided to the adoptive parent(s) for children with special needs.

International Adoption

International adoption is when a child is adopted through a private agency which facilitates an intercountry adoption. Some agencies focus on only one country, while others work with many countries and can offer children of various backgrounds. When adopting internationally, the adoptive parent(s) must meet the requirements of both the child's home country and the U.S. Citizenship and Immigration Services. The process can be more complex than domestic adoption options, as factors such as the age of the child, medical care, and adoptive parent criteria vary greatly from country to country.

Accordingly, people considering adoption have a wide range of options. It is often said that adopting is both a legal process and an emotional one. There are a tremendous amount of resources available to educate and support you through the process. Please see Appendix B for more information.

82. Is it possible to adopt if you have a history of cancer?

Yes, it is possible to adopt even if you have had cancer; however, most adoption agencies will consider your medical history and may require you to be a certain number of years out from your treatment and/or require a letter from your doctor about your health status. In addition, many foreign countries have their own specific requirements addressing the potential parent(s)' health, and thus, agencies working with those countries are often limited by strict rules. It is important to choose an agency and country that is open to working with cancer survivors.

83. What are the average costs of adoption?

There are many factors that influence the cost of adoption. The adoption fee should include the costs of doing a **home study**, preadoptive counseling, identification of a child for your family, placement fees, and postplacement visits.

The average cost of adopting a child in the United States varies according to the type of placement:

It is important to choose an agency and country that is open to working with cancer survivors.

Home study

Process where an adoption caseworker interviews potential parents to evaluate whether they are qualified to adopt according to the guidelines of the agency, state, or country where they are adopting from. Usually background checks, financial reviews, and at least one home visit are part of the process.

- Independent adoption ranges from $8,000 to $30,000 or more.
- Private agency adoption ranges from $4,000 to $30,000 or more.
- Public agency adoptions, where children are adopted from the foster care system, range from $0 to $2,500.
- International adoption ranges from $7,000 to $30,000 or more.

In the United States, there is an adoption tax credit that will allow you to take a credit of up to up to $10,960 in 2006 for the adoption of a child.

In the United States, there is an adoption tax credit that will allow you to take a credit of up to up to $10,960 in 2006 for the adoption of a child (the tax credit amount changes annually—please ask your tax advisor how much you may be able to deduct). Some companies also offer a leave of absence similar to maternity/paternity leave, as well as reimbursements for certain expenses. More information about tax credits, employer benefits, adoption loans, and governmental subsidies is available through the National Adoption Information Clearinghouse at http://naic.acf.hhs.gov.

84. How long does adoption take?

The average time it takes to adopt a child depends on the type of adoption you select. Adopting a child almost always requires a waiting period and a home study. In the United States, if you want to adopt a Caucasian infant, it may take up to 1 to 5 years from the time the home study is completed. Applicants wishing to adopt children of other ethnicities may have a shorter wait, sometimes less than 6 months. The process is much faster if you are adopting an older child or a child with special needs. Finally, international adoptions may take a year or more. For any type of adoption, even after a child is found, you may have to wait weeks or months while final arrangements are made.

PART TWELVE

Children After Cancer

Will my children be at risk for birth defects
because of my cancer treatments?

Will my children have a higher risk of
getting cancer because I had it?

What is preimplantation genetic diagnosis (PGD)?
How is it used for cancer survivors?

85. Will my children be at risk for birth defects because of my cancer treatments?

This is one of the most common questions asked by cancer survivors. There has not been a vast amount of research done on the subject, but what has been done is very reassuring. The rate of birth defects in children born to cancer survivors (who have been exposed to chemo and radiation) is the same as the general public, 2% to 3%.

The rate of birth defects in children born to cancer survivors (who have been exposed to chemo and radiation) is the same as the general public, 2% to 3%.

86. Will my children have a higher risk of getting cancer because I had it?

In most cases, having a cancer diagnosis itself does not appear to increase your chances of having a child who will develop cancer. Your child's risk of developing cancer appears to be the same as that of the general public, unless you have a genetically linked cancer or cancer syndrome. A small percent of cancers of the breast, ovary, colon, pancreas, and kidney may be hereditary. The list of truly genetic cancers is constantly being updated. Check with your doctor or a genetic counselor to understand better whether your cancer is hereditary.

Preimplantation genetic diagnosis (PGD)

A technique used during the in vitro fertilization process to test embryos for genetic disorders before their transfer to the uterus. PGD makes it possible for individuals with serious inherited disorders to decrease the risk of having a child who is affected by the disorder.

If you do have a genetic cancer and the gene that causes it is known, you may be able to use a test called **preimplantation genetic diagnosis** (PGD) to screen your embryos for that gene to avoid passing it on. For more information about PGD, please see Question 87.

87. What is preimplantation genetic diagnosis? How is it used for cancer survivors?

Preimplantation genetic diagnosis (PGD) is a technique used during the IVF process to test embryos for genetic disorders. After embryos are created, they are allowed to mature in the laboratory for 3 days. After the embryos reach a certain stage of development, a single cell can be removed from the embryo and tested for the presence of certain genetic disorders. The embryos that do not contain the disorder can then be transferred to your uterus or frozen for future use. The embryos that contain the genetic defect can be discarded or donated to research. Alternatively, some couples may also choose to implant embryos with known genetic disorders. For example, if the genetic disorder will result in a predisposition for a disease, couples may still choose to implant those embryos. Currently, PGD testing is available for these cancer predispositions:

- Breast Cancer 1 Gene
- Breast Cancer 2 Gene
- Familial Adenomatous Polyposis
- Gorlin Syndrome (Basel Cell Nevus Carcinoma Syndrome)
- Lynch Syndrome (Hereditary Nonpolyposis Colorectal Cancer)
- Li-Fraumeni Syndrome
- Multiple Endocrine Neoplasia
- Neurofibromatosis Type 1
- Neurofibromatosis Type 2
- Rhabdoid Predisposition Syndrome
- Retinoblastoma
- Tuberous sclerosis Type 1
- Tuberous sclerosis Type 2
- Von Hippel-Lindau Disease

PGD makes it possible for individuals with serious genetic disorders to decrease the risk of having a child who is affected by the disorder. It is now possible to use this technique to help decrease the risk of passing on some cancer-related genes to your offspring. The list of detectable disorders is constantly being updated. Check with your reproductive specialist to see whether PGD can be used to identify the specific genetic disorder that you are concerned about. The average cost of PGD is $5,000 per cycle.

PART THIRTEEN

Financial Issues

Does insurance cover fertility preservation
or assisted reproduction treatments?

Are there financial assistance programs available?

At that point, again being single, I had no one steady in my life; the thought of using donated sperm was at the time totally preposterous. On top of all of that, none of the services, either my visits to the fertility specialist, any tests, the treatments, the embryo storage, the "thawing," or any future options, was covered by insurance. Because the process was considered a fertility issue versus a side effect from cancer treatment, it was not covered by insurance. All of the other side effects from cancer treatment were covered by insurance, except for fertility treatment. All of this would have been out of pocket, and there was no way we or my family could afford it. I decided . . . to let fate take its course.

—Amy, Non-Hodgkin's Lymphoma

88. Does insurance cover fertility preservation or assisted reproduction treatments?

Currently, there are 13 states with laws mandating some level of insurance coverage for infertility diagnosis and treatment. There are no laws that directly address coverage for fertility preservation or cancer-related infertility.

There are no laws that directly address coverage for fertility preservation or cancer-related infertility.

Most plans that offer coverage define infertility as the inability to conceive after 1 year of unprotected intercourse. Accordingly, a cancer patient may not meet that definition, as the patient is not usually known to be infertile at the time of diagnosis. As a result, even if you have fertility coverage, you may be denied benefits because you do not meet the insurer's definition of "infertility."

Some patients with existing fertility coverage have petitioned their insurance company explaining their extenuating circumstances. In some cases, benefits have been provided.

89. Are there financial assistance programs available?

Many different financial resources are available that may be of assistance to you.

Many different financial resources are available that may be of assistance to you.

Insurance Coverage

To learn more about possible insurance coverage for fertility treatments, consult the following resources:

- **American Fertility Association**
  www.theafa.org.

- **American Society for Reproductive Medicine**
  www.ASRM.org.

- **INCIID**
  www.inciid.org.

- **National Conference of State Legislators**
  http://www.ncsl.org/programs/health/50infert.htm
  50 State Summary of State Laws Related to Insurance Coverage for Infertility Therapy

- **RESOLVE: The National Infertility Association**
  www.resolve.org

Financing

Many fertility clinics offer their own financing programs for their patients. We encourage you to speak with a professional in your healthcare provider's office to learn more about their financing and shared risk options. Some of these are as follows:

- **Capital One Healthcare Finance**
  www.capitalonehealthcarefinance.com/fertility
  Available through Capital One, Inc., the Healthcare Finance program provides low, fixed-rate loans to cover fertility treatments. If your doctor is not registered for the program, a Capital One sales consultant can contact your doctor to help him/her register.

- **Care Credit**
  www.carecredit.com/
  Care Credit is a flexible patient/client payment program, specifically designed for healthcare expenses.

Financial Issues

They offer a full range of no-interest and extended-payment plans for treatment fees.

- **Extend Fertility**
  www.extendfertility.com
  Financing options for egg freezing are available. Extend Fertility works with a network of fertility centers to offer egg freezing services.

- **IntegraMed Financial Services Program**
  www.integramed.com/inmdweb/content/cons/
  financing.jsp
  IntegraMed Financial Services offers convenient, low-interest healthcare financing for any type of infertility treatment. Infertility treatments, as well as medications, are eligible for coverage under a simple monthly payment plan.

Shared Risk Programs

Shared risk program

Payment option for people when their insurance does not cover in vitro fertilization (IVF). The patient pays a fixed up-front cost for a set number of IVF attempts. If there is no successful pregnancy after the IVF attempts, the money is refunded.

Many fertility clinics offer their own **shared risk programs** for their patients. These programs generally offer refunds if pregnancy is not achieved within a certain number of cycles. Because the guarantees are tied to the program, they are not really applicable for fertility preservation. We encourage you to speak with a professional in your healthcare providers' office to learn more about their financing and shared risk options:

- **Advanced Reproductive Care, Inc. (ARC)**
  www.arcfertility.com/
  ARC is a nationwide network of reproductive endocrinologists and fertility programs that offer treatment packages, financing programs, and a refund guarantee that provides a return of up to 100% of your medicals costs if treatment is unsuccessful.

- **IntegraMed Shared Risk Refund Program**
  www.integramed.com/inmdweb/content/cons/shared.
  jsp
  The IntegraMed Shared Risk Refund Program offers a six-cycle treatment package and minimizes the finan-

cial risk by fixing the cost of treatment and providing a significant refund if treatment is not successful. You must be treated in one of their participating fertility centers, which are available nationwide.

Financial Assistance Programs: Fertility Preservation

- **Fertile Hope's "Sharing Hope" Program**
  www.fertilehope.org
  Through Sharing Hope, Fertile Hope offers assistance for qualified men and women applicants by providing discounted sperm banking services, access to fertility medications donated by EMD Serono, Inc., and discounted egg and embryo freezing services from reproductive endocrinologists from across the country. The Sharing Hope program does not itself grant financial contributions but instead has aligned with key organizations to make egg, embryo, and sperm freezing more accessible. Women must be treated by a participating Sharing Hope fertility center, and men must use the services of our partnering **cryobank**.

- **Partnership for Families Program**
  http://cms.clevelandclinic.org/obgyn/body.cfm?id=86&oTopID=86
  The Partnership for Families Program at the Cleveland Clinic Fertility Center at Beachwood provides funding for the first cycle of embryo or egg freezing for qualified patients.

Financial Assistance Programs: Fertility Medications

The following programs may be able to provide donated fertility medications:

- **Bravelle HEART (Helping Expand Access to Reproductive Therapy) Program**
  http://www.ferringfertility.com/ourproducts/heart/index.asp
  Sponsored by Ferring Pharmaceuticals, this program provides infertility patients with five free vials of

Through Sharing Hope, Fertile Hope offers assistance for qualified men and women applicants by providing discounted sperm banking services, access to fertility medications donated by EMD Serono, Inc., and discounted egg and embryo freezing services from reproductive endocrinologists from across the country.

Financial Issues

Cryobank
A facility where tissues such as sperm, oocytes, and embryos are stored in the frozen state.

Bravelle as part of a prescription of 20 or more vials. Bravelle HEART is only available at participating pharmacies.

- **FertilityAssist**
  http://www.fertilitylifelines.com/paying/fertilityassist/index.jsp?intcmp=FA
  This program offers EMD Serono, Inc. fertility medications free of charge to eligible patients through Freedom Fertility Pharmacy for the third cycle if the patient has not been successful after the prior two attempts.

- **Organon Fertility Patient Assistance Program**
  This program provides financial assistance for Organon medications. Contact your physician for more information.

Financial Assistance Programs: Achieving Pregnancy

The following programs assist with the cost associated with achieving pregnancy.

- **INCIID**
  http://www.inciid.org/
  The InterNational Council of Infertility Information Dissemination offers a program titled "From INCIID the Heart" designed to provide free in vitro fertilization to those without insurance who have both financial and medical need for the procedure.

- **New York State Fertility Demonstration Project**
  http://www.health.state.ny.us/nysdoh/infertility/index.htm
  In June 2002, legislation was signed in New York that authorized $10 million to subsidize high-level infertility treatments for privately insured women whose insurance did not cover these procedures. The Department of Health invited select infertility providers statewide to participate in the program.

- **Partnership for Families Program**
  http://cms.clevelandclinic.org/obgyn/body.
  cfm?id=158&oTopID=86
  The Partnership for Families program at the Cleveland
  Clinic Fertility Center at Beachwood provides funding
  for a second cycle of in vitro fertilization to couples
  who otherwise could not afford another try.

Research & Trials

Specific experimental procedures may be available at no or
low cost as part of research studies. For more information
and a list of research on current trials, please visit www.
fertilehope.org.

PART FOURTEEN

Emotional and Social Concerns

What strategies can help me cope with fertility in addition to cancer?

Are there professionals who can help me cope with the emotional aspects of cancer and fertility?

If I am dating, how do I talk about this?

More . . .

Initially, I was devastated when I learned that I might not be able to have children. I was single and the one thought that kept entering my mind was that no one would ever want to marry me if I couldn't have children. I was scared at the thought of being single forever and dying alone.

—Adrianne, Chronic Myelogenous Leukemia

90. What strategies can help me cope with fertility in addition to cancer?

Many cancer patients feel like cancer-related infertility is a double blow.

Many cancer patients feel like cancer-related infertility is a double blow. Feelings of anger, denial, depression, resentment, blame, and lack of control are common and understandable. Here are a few tips that may help you cope with this wide spectrum of emotions:

- Recognize this as true loss.
- Accept your emotions.
- Do not blame yourself or your partner.
- Work as a team with you partner, family, and/or health-care professionals.
- Educate yourself.
- Set limits on what you are willing to do and how much you are willing to pay.
- Get support.
- Avoid upsetting activities (e.g., baby showers).
- Balance hope with reality.
- Take care of yourself.
- Talk to friends and family.

Do what feels right for you as you work through the challenges of cancer-related infertility.

It is alright to grieve and be angry about the loss. It is not fair, and it is not something that you need to be stoic about or be made to believe that is a small price to pay for your life.

—Karen, Pediatric Rhabdomyosarcoma

91. Are there professionals who can help me cope with the emotional aspects of cancer and fertility?

There are many resources available to help you cope with the emotional aspects of cancer-related infertility. A few include the following:

- Nurses
- Social workers
- Mental health professionals
- Support groups
- Chat rooms/message boards
- Mentor—someone who has been there and understands

You are not alone. Many people have struggled with many of the same issues you are struggling with and there are a lot of resources out there to help.

It has had a tremendous effect on my life as well as many others. I now understand how much it can affect someone's life and self esteem to not be able to have children.

—Jamie, Neuroblastoma

92. If I am dating, how do I talk about this?

As with any personal medical situation, the best time to share this information with a prospective new boyfriend or girlfriend is when you are comfortable. Some resources say never talk about it on the first date or offer more strict guidelines on what is best, but in the end, only you know what is right for you.

If you are having a hard time dating after cancer, it may help to know that many survivors have shared the same struggles and have overcome their difficulties. Some have said that one of the most challenging things about dating after cancer is figuring out when to share their experience and disclose long-term side effects such as infertility. Some ways to tell

If you are having a hard time dating after cancer, it may help to know that many survivors have shared the same struggles and have overcome their difficulties.

the people you date that you are a survivor and/or may have fertility complications include the following:

- Waiting to tell them because you want to get to know them better before you share something that you feel is very personal
- Telling them right away to get it over with and see how they react
- Taking things on a case-by-case basis and telling someone when the moment feels right

All of these approaches are valid. Thus, you must decide what feels comfortable to you. You have a special story to tell and, when you are ready, you can feel proud to talk about it with others.

Because my entire dating/single life has been lived after treatment when I've been in Premature Ovarian Failure (POF), I have experienced firsthand the difficulty in balancing a single life with infertility. Should I tell him? When should I tell? I always told my serious boyfriends and every one of them reacted in an understanding and supportive way; I never had a bad experience. I told them when I knew that it was turning into a serious and trustworthy relationship, but before it had gotten more than a few months into it. I didn't want to withhold something that is understandably important to so many people, but at the same time, I don't think it defines who I am as a person so much that I would want to tell someone I'm interested in immediately.

—Karen, Pediatric Rhabdomyosarcoma

93. If I froze sperm, eggs, embryos, or tissue before cancer treatments but I never use them or I have some left over after completing my family, what do I do with them?

If you choose not to use your frozen sperm, eggs, embryos, or tissue, you generally have three choices on what to do with the tissue:

- Discard them
- Donate them to research
- Donate them to another person or couple who is trying to have a child

This is a very personal decision for you. Generally, before freezing any of these tissues, your fertility specialist will ask you to think about what you would like done in the event of your death, divorce, or other unforeseen circumstances.

94. If I have children with donor sperm, eggs, or embryos or if I use a gestational surrogate, how do I explain this to my family and friends?

There is no right answer to this question. Some experts believe that this is a topic that you should explain to your children early on, with increasing details as the child matures and can understand them. Most agree that this information should not be kept as a secret from your child for fear that it could traumatize the child and shake their sense of identity when they do learn of the special circumstances of their birth. There are several books, fact sheets, and Web site resources available to help you determine what works best for your family.

PART FIFTEEN

Finding the Services You Need

How do I find a reputable sperm bank?

How do I find a reproductive specialist
or fertility center?

How do I find donor sperm?

More...

Be your own advocate! This is a very difficult time; there are many things to consider, but you know what is best for you. The doctors have a focus, and it's why they are good at what they do. You need to advocate for yourself, however, so that you know all of the options available to you and you can make the best decisions. Also, don't underestimate your ability to learn what you need to know to make those decisions. Read and do research and become an expert on the issues related to your cancer. You will be stronger for it and will be a valuable resource to someone else in the future.

—Debbie, Breast Cancer

95. How do I find a reputable sperm bank?

The best first step to finding a sperm bank is to ask your doctor for a referral.

The best first step to finding a sperm bank is to ask your doctor for a referral. Additional resources that may be able to help you find one that best suits your needs include the following:

- American Association of Tissue Banks: www.aatb.org
- Fertile Hope: www.fertilehope.org
- Sperm Bank Directory: www.spermbankdirectory.com

If there is not a sperm bank in your area, you may also bank your sperm using a special kit that is mailed to a sperm bank.

If there is not a sperm bank in your area, you may also bank your sperm using a special kit that is mailed to a sperm bank. Some national sperm banks have kits that they will send to your home or your doctor's office. You follow the directions and deposit your sperm into the container and solution they provide. The solution protects the sperm so that it can be mailed back to the sperm bank overnight and stored for future use. It is important to know that some of the sperm do not survive the process. Banking at the sperm bank is more successful in terms of the percentage of sperm that survive.

96. How do I find a reproductive specialist or fertility center?

Choosing a fertility center is an important decision. The following are some factors you may want to consider when choosing your fertility doctor, center, or service:

- Success/pregnancy rates
- Qualifications and experience of doctors and other personnel
- Types of services offered, especially if you are looking for experimental procedures
- Cost
- Convenience
- Recommendations and reputation
- Friendliness of staff and physicians
- Environment (peaceful, respectful, comfortable, etc.)

Pregnancy rates for each clinic are published online by both the Centers for Disease Control (CDC) and the Society for Assisted Reproductive Technology (SART). The following links may help you find and compare success rates:

- **CDC Assisted Reproductive Technology Home Page**
  http://www.cdc.gov/ART/

- **SART Summary Report (National Average)**
  https://www.sartcorsonline.com/rptCSR_PublicMult-Year.aspx?ClinicPKID=0

- **SART Searchable Database of Centers with Individual Reports**
  http://www.sart.org/find_frm.html

These numbers are 2 to 3 years old and can sometimes be reported differently by different centers; thus, these figures should not be the only factor that you consider.

As a cancer patient or survivor, you may have special concerns when choosing a clinic. For example, if you are looking to preserve your fertility, you may need to begin your reproductive treatments quickly, and you will need to work with a doctor who understands this. Many fertility preservation technologies, such as testicular tissue freezing, ovarian tissue freezing and egg freezing, are still considered experimental, and only a limited number of fertility clinics have experience with these services.

Many fertility preservation technologies, such as testicular tissue freezing, ovarian tissue freezing and egg freezing, are still considered experimental, and only a limited number of fertility clinics have experience with these services.

The following are sample questions that may help you make an informed decision:

- What procedures do you offer?
- How much experience do you have in these procedures and what are your success rates? (e.g., How many babies born?)
- Do your physicians have experience working with cancer patients?
- How long do I have to wait for an appointment?
- What are your criteria for seeing patients (e.g., age limits and single versus married versus partnered)?
- What screening tests are required?
- What is the time commitment?
- Does the program meet and follow American Society for Reproductive Medicine guidelines?
- Does the program report its results to the Society for Assisted Reproductive Technology (SART) Registry and the Centers for Disease Control (CDC)?
- Is the program a member of the SART?
- How many physicians will be involved in my care?
- Are your physicians board certified in reproductive endocrinology and in good medical standing?
- What types of counseling and support services are available?
- Do you have an outline of the costs of the tests and procedures I may need?
- Do you accept insurance?
- What are your available payment options?
- Is staff accessible to answer questions about treatment, forms, or payment?
- What are the ongoing storage costs of tissues (sperm, eggs, etc.)?

Spend the time you need to select a program that best meets your unique needs.

Do the research. Push your doctors. Don't be afraid to take time! In many cases, you do have time to evaluate your risks and options before having to start treatment.

—Heidi, Ewing's Sarcoma

97. How do I find donor sperm?

Currently, in the United States, sperm banks are not regulated. There are voluntary guidelines issued by the American Society of Reproductive Medicine (ASRM) as well as the American Association of Tissue Banks (AATB). There are some federal and state laws for the banks to follow, but it is generally recommended that you work with a bank that is fully accredited by the AATB.

Sample questions you may want to ask a bank include:

- Are your donors are tested for HIV-1, HIV-2, hepatitis B and C, htlV-1, and CMV?
- Are your donors tested at the time of the deposit as well as 6 months later, and is the sperm quarantined during that time?
- How old are your donors (e.g., is there an age limit)?
- How many pregnancies do you allow per donor?
- Do you keep in touch with your donors?
- Do you have records of any birth defects or health problems in the children born from your donors?

Costs vary greatly from center to center, and thus, during your evaluation, you may want to inquire about prices as well.

98. How do I find donor eggs and embryos?

You can find an anonymous egg donor through your fertility clinic or an agency, or you can use a known donor such as a relative or friend. If you choose an anonymous donor, you will usually be able to choose her based on physical characteristics, ethnic background, educational record, and occupation. Most donors are between 21 and 29 years old and have undergone psychological, medical, and genetic screening. Some centers do more extensive tests and background checks than others.

Recently, the first donor egg bank opened, which means that it is also possible to buy donor eggs from a third-party agency, not just your fertility clinic. This option is new and controversial, mainly because the eggs donated to the egg bank are frozen, not fresh. As discussed in the egg-freezing section, the technique is still experimental, and the success rates are not as high as the traditional method.

If you choose to use donor embryos, you can either pick unrelated egg and sperm donors or use a frozen embryo donated by a couple that had extras. You can work with your fertility clinic or a third-party donor embryo agency.

As discussed in Question 60, there are Food and Drug Administration (FDA) regulations that require clinics using donor eggs and embryos to perform screening for certain infectious disease as well as meet other storage and reporting standards. The ASRM also has guidelines around the screening and compensation of donors. When selecting a clinic or agency to work with, it is recommended that you ask whether they comply with these regulations and guidelines.

99. How do I choose an adoption agency?

Choosing an adoption agency requires research and networking to help ensure that you find an agency that meets your needs throughout the process. A few tips that may be helpful include the following:

- Gather as much information as possible.
- Evaluate agencies based on the information gathered.
- Ask a lot of questions.
- Compare services offered by various agencies.
- Network with others.

- Understand the fee structures: what is charged and when it is due.
- Make sure the agency and its employees are licensed professionals.
- Find out how long the agency has been in operation and how many children it has placed.
- Request professional affiliations and references.
- Look out for red flags.

Take the necessary time to select an adoption agency carefully, as it may save you a lot of unnecessary stress and loss down the road. Moreover, choosing the right agency will help improve the chances of a smooth process and successful outcome for your family.

100. How do I find a surrogate?

Generally, couples work with their fertility clinic or an agency to find a surrogate, although some couples arrange this on their own. Surrogacy arrangements are contractual agreements between the couple and the surrogate. Laws governing surrogacy vary widely, and thus, it is advisable to get legal counsel before entering this type of agreement.

There are many legal, ethical, and practical issues surround surrogacy that should be considered carefully. For couples who are thinking about surrogacy, the following questions may be helpful:

- How long has the surrogacy program been in operation?
- What are the costs of surrogacy (traditional, gestational, or donor)? What is the fee payment structure? How are the surrogate's expenses handled? Is there a cap on these expenses?
- What type of legal counsel is offered to the surrogate and the couple? Does this include the drawing up of contracts?

Take the necessary time to select an adoption agency carefully, as it may save you a lot of unnecessary stress and loss down the road.

There are many legal, ethical, and practical issues surround surrogacy that should be considered carefully.

Finding the Services You Need

113

- If the surrogate does not get pregnant over a certain number of cycles, what is the clinic's policy regarding refund of fee paid?
- In the event that the contract is not honored, what are the financial obligations for the couple? In the event that the surrogate has a pregnancy loss, what are the financial obligations for the couple?
- How are the surrogates chosen? By the agency? By the couple?
- How are the surrogates screened? What does medical screening include? Is there psychological screening? Is the surrogate's partner screened?
- What type of emotional support does the program offer for the couple? For the surrogate? Counseling or support groups?
- How many babies have been born through the clinic's surrogacy programs?
- To what extent is contact between the surrogate and the couple encouraged? Required? By letter, meeting face to face, ongoing?
- Can the couple be involved in doctor's visits with the surrogate, such as ultrasounds?
- Who makes the medical decisions during the pregnancy, such as the decision to have amniocentesis or to terminate if necessary? What if the surrogate does not want to undergo a procedure that the couple wants done?
- Can the couple be present in the delivery room at the birth?
- Does the program maintain a referral listing of previous client couples?

Appendix A

Appendix A includes the following tables:

- Males—Risk of Azoospermia
- Male Options for Parenthood
- Females—Risk of Amenorrhea
- Female Options for Parenthood

Table 1   Males—Risk of Azoospermia

Degree of Risk	Treatment Protocol	Type of Cancer Used For
High Risk Prolonged azoospermia post-treatment	Total Body Irradiation (TBI)	bone marrow transplant/stem cell transplant (BMT/SCT)
	Testicular Radiation Dose (> 2.5 Gy) in adults	testicular cancer, acute lymphoblastic leukemia (ALL), non-Hodgkin lymphoma (NHL)
	Testicular Radiation Dose ≥ 6 Gy in child	ALL, NHL, sarcoma, germ cell tumors
	Protocols containing procarbazine: COPP, MOPP, MVPP, ChIVPP, ChIVPP/EVA, MOPP/ABVD, COPP/ABVD	Hodgkin lymphoma
	Alkylating chemotherapy for transplant conditioning (Cyclophosphamide, Busulfan, melphalan)	BMT/SCT
	Any alkylating agent (e.g., procarbazine, nitrogen mustard, cyclophosphamide) + TBI, pelvic radiation, or testicular radiation	Testicular Cancer, BMT/SCT, ALL, NHL, sarcoma, neuroblastoma, Hodgkin lymphoma
	Cyclophosphamide >7.5 g/m^2	sarcoma, NHL, neuroblastoma, ALL
	Cranial/brain radiation ≥ 40 Gy	Brain tumor

(continued)

Table 1   Males—Risk of Azoospermia (continued)

Degree of Risk	Treatment Protocol	Type of Cancer Used For
Intermediate Risk Prolonged azoospermia not common at standard dose	BEP × 2–4 cycles (bleomycin, etoposide, cisplatin)	testicular cancer
	Cumulative cisplatin dose < 400 mg/m²	testicular cancer
	Cumulative carboplatin dose </= 2g/m²	testicular cancer
	Testicular Radiation Dose 1–6Gy	Scatter from abdominal/pelvic radiation for Wilms tumor, neuroblastoma
Low Risk **Temporary** azoospermia post-treatment	Non-alkylating chemotherapy: ABVD, OEPA, NOVP, CHOP, COP	Hodgkin lymphoma, NHL
	Testicular Radiation Dose (0.2–0.7 Gy)	testicular cancer
Very Low/ No Risk No effects on sperm production	Testicular Radiation Dose (< 0.2 Gy)	
	Interferon-a	multiple cancers
	Radioactive Iodine	thyroid
Unknown Risk	Irinotecan	colon
	Bevacizumab (Avastin)	colon, non-small cell lung
	Cetuximab (Erbitux)	colon, head & neck
	Erlotinib (Tarceva)	non-small cell lung, pancreatic
	Imatinib (Gleevec)	chronic myeloid leukemia (CML), gastrointestinal stromal tumor (GIST)

© Fertile Hope 2007. Reprinted with permission.

Table 2: Male Options

Method	Timing	Definition	Medical Status	Time Requirement	Success Rates	Average Cost	Age	Special Considerations
Sperm Banking (Masturbation)	Before treatment	Sperm is obtained through masturbation, then frozen	Standard	Outpatient procedure	Generally High The most established technique for men	$1,500 for 3 samples stored for 3 years Future storage fees average $500/year	After Puberty	Deposits can be made every 24 hours
Sperm Banking (Alternative Collection Methods)	Before treatment	Freezing sperm obtained through testicular aspiration, extraction, or electroejaculation under sedation	Experimental	Outpatient procedures	If sperm is obtained, success rates are similar to standard sperm banking	Varies greatly based on collection method	After Puberty	Can be considered if male cannot ejaculate

(continued)

Table 2: Male Options (continued)

Method	Timing	Definition	Medical Status	Time Requirement	Success Rates	Average Cost	Age	Special Considerations
Testicular Tissue Freezing	Before treatment	Tissue is obtained through biopsy and frozen for either reimplantation or in vitro maturation of sperm cells	Experimental	Outpatient procedure	No available human success rates	$500–$2,500 for surgery $300–$1,000 for freezing tissue Storage fees average $100–500/year	Before and After Puberty	Still experimental, but may be the only option for pre-pubescent boys
Testicular Sperm Extraction	Before or after treatment	Use of biopsy to obtain individual sperm from testicular tissue	Standard	Outpatient procedure	30–70% in post-pubescent patients	$6,000–$16,000 (in addition to costs for IVF)	After Puberty	Important to work with a center that can freeze any sperm found during biopsy

(continued)

Table 2: Male Options (continued)

Method	Timing	Definition	Medical Status	Time Requirement	Success Rates	Average Cost	Age	Special Considerations
Radiation Shielding of Gonads	During treatment	Use of shielding to reduce the dose of radiation delivered to the testes	Standard	In conjunction with radiation treatments	Possible with select radiation fields and anatomy	Generally included in the cost of radiation treatments	Before and After Puberty	Expertise required; Does not protect against effects of chemotherapy
Donor Sperm	After treatment	Sperm donated by a man for artificial insemination	Standard	Readily available for purchase	50–80%	$200–$500 per vial (in addition to costs for IUI or IVF)	After Puberty	Patient can choose donor from wide range of characteristics
Adoption	After treatment	Legal proceeding that creates a parent-child relation	Standard	Varies depending on the type of adoption	Varies Greatly	$2,500–$35,000	After Puberty	Can be difficult for cancer survivors given health history

© Fertile Hope 2007. Reprinted with permission.

Table 3: Females—Risk of Amenorrhea

This table represents a compilation of both clinical experience and the findings in the current literature of the impact of common cancer treatments on menstruation. Generally, studies have not focused on other measures of reproductive capacity, such as hormone levels or follicle counts. Most studies have measured menstruation, which may not accurately reflect reproductive capacity.

Degree of Risk	Treatment Protocol	Type of Cancer Used For
High Risk >80% of women develop amenorrhea post-treatment	Whole abdominal or pelvic radiation doses $\geq$ 6 Gy in adult women	
	Whole abdominal or pelvic radiation doses $\geq$ 15 Gy in pre-pubertal girls $\geq$ 10 Gy in post-pubertal girls	Wilms' tumor, neuroblastoma, sarcoma, Hodgkin lymphoma
	TBI radiation doses	bone marrow transplant/ stem cell transplant (BMT/ SCT)
	CMF, CEF, CAF x 6 cycles in women 40+	breast cancer
	Cyclophosphamide 5 g/m² in women 40+	multiple cancers
	Cyclophosphamide 7.5 g/m² in girls < 20	non-Hodgkin lymphoma (NHL), neuroblastoma, acute lymphoblastic leukemia (ALL), sarcoma
	Alkylating chemotherapy (e.g., cyclophosphamide, busulfan, melaphan) conditioning for transplant	BMT/SCT
	Any alkylating agent (e.g., cyclophosphamide, ifosfamide, busulfan, BCNU, CCNU) + TBI or pelvic radiation	BMT/SCT, ovarian cancer, sarcoma, neuroblastoma, Hodgkin lymphoma
	Protocols containing procarbazine: MOPP, MVPP, COPP, ChIVPP, ChIVPP/EVA, BEACOPP, MOPP/ABVD, COPP/ABVD	Hodgkin lymphoma
	Cranial/brain radiation $\geq$40 Gy	brain tumor
Intermediate Risk ~30-70% of women develop amenorrhea post-treatment	CMF or CEF or CAF women 30-39	breast cancer
	AC in women 40+	breast cancer
	Whole abdominal or pelvic radiation 10-<15 Gy in prepubertal girls	Wilms' tumor
	Whole abdominal or pelvic radiation 5-<10 Gy in postpubertal girls	Wilms' tumor, neuroblastoma
	Spinal radiation $\geq$25 Gy	spinal tumor, brain tumor, neuroblastoma, relapsed ALL or NHL

(continued)

Table 3: Females—Risk of Amenorrhea (continued)

Degree of Risk	Treatment Protocol	Type of Cancer Used For
Low Risk <20% of women develop amenorrhea post-treatment	AC in women 30–39	breast cancer
	CMF, CEF, or CAF × 6 cycles in women under 30	breast cancer
	Non-alkylating chemotherapy: ABVD, CHOP, COP	Hodgkin lymphoma, NHL
	AC (anthracycline, cytarabine)	acute myeloid leukemia (AML)
	Multi-agent therapies	ALL
Very Low/ No Risk Negligible effect on menses	MF (methotrexate, 5-FU)	breast cancer
	Vincristine (used in multi-agent therapies)	leukemia, Hodgkin, lymphoma, NHL, neuroblastoma, rhabdomyosarcoma, Wilms' tumor , Kaposi's sarcoma
	Radioactive Iodine	thyroid cancer
Unknown Risk	Paclitaxel, Docetaxel (Taxanes used in AC protocols)	breast cancer
	Oxaliplatin	ovarian cancer
	Irinotecan	colon cancer
	Bevacizumab (Avastin)	colon, non-small cell lung
	Cetuximab (Erbitux)	colon, head & neck
	Trastuzamab (Herceptin)	breast cancer
	Erlotinib (Tarceva)	non-small cell lung, pancreatic
	Imatinib (Gleevec)	chronic myeloid leukemia (CML), gastrointestinal stromal tumor (GIST)

Table 4: Female Options

Method	Timing	Definition	Medical Status	Time Requirement	Success Rates	Cost	Pubertal Status	Special Considerations
Embryo Freezing	Before or after treatment	Harvesting eggs, in vitro fertilization and freezing of embryos for later implantation	Standard	10-14 days of ovarian stimulation from onset of menses Outpatient surgical procedure	Varies based on age and expertise of center Approximately 40% per 3 embryos transferred in women under 35; lower in older women Thousands born	$8,000/ cycle, plus $,3500–$5,000 for medications Long term storage fees average $500/year Additional costs apply when pregnancy is sought	After Puberty	Requires partner or donor sperm Experimental protocols exist for hormone-sensitive cancers

(continued)

Table 4: Female Options (continued)

Method	Timing	Definition	Medical Status	Time Requirement	Success Rates	Cost	Pubertal Status	Special Considerations
Egg Freezing	Before or after treatment	Harvesting and freezing of unfertilized eggs	Experimental	10–14 days of ovarian stimulation from the onset menses Outpatient surgical procedure	Approximately 21.6% per embryo transfer Approximately 3–4 times lower than embryo freezing 200+ live births reported to date	$8,000/cycle, plus $3,500–$5,000 for medications Long term storage fees average $500/year Additional costs apply when pregnancy is sought	After Puberty	Maybe desirable for single women or those opposed to embryo creation Experimental protocols exist for hormone-sensitive cancers

(continued)

Table 4: Female Options (continued)

Method	Timing	Definition	Medical Status	Time Requirement	Success Rates	Cost	Pubertal Status	Special Considerations
Ovarian Tissue Freezing	Before or after treatment	Freezing of ovarian tissue and reimplantation after cancer treatment	Experimental	Outpatient surgical procedure	Case reports of 2 live births reported	$12,000/ procedure

Long term storage averages $500/year

Additional costs apply when tissue is re-implanted or pregnancy is sought | Before or After Puberty | Not suitable when risk of ovarian metastases is high

May be the only preservation option for pre-pubescent girls |
| Ovarian Transposition | Before treatment | Surgical repositioning of ovaries away from the radiation field | Standard | Outpatient procedure | Approximately 50% due to altered ovarian blood flow and scattered radiation | Unknown

Generally covered by insurance | Before or After Puberty | Expertise required |

(continued)

Table 4: Female Options (continued)

Method	Timing	Definition	Medical Status	Time Requirement	Success Rates	Cost	Pubertal Status	Special Considerations
Radiation Shielding of Gonads	During treatment	Use of shielding to reduce scatter radiation to the reproductive organs	Standard	In conjunction with radiation treatments	Only possible with selected radiation fields and anatomy	Generally included in cost of radiation	Before and After Puberty	Expertise required Does not protect against effects of chemotherapy
Trachelectomy	During treatment	Surgical removal of the cervix with preservation of the uterus	Standard	Inpatient surgical procedure	No evidence of higher cancer recurrence rates in appropriate candidates	Generally included in the cost of cancer treatment	After Puberty	Limited to early stage cervical cancer Offered at a limited number of centers

(continued)

125

Table 4: Female Options (continued)

Method	Timing	Definition	Medical Status	Time Requirement	Success Rates	Cost	Pubertal Status	Special Considerations
Ovarian Suppression	During treatment	Use of GnRH Analogs or Antagonists to protect ovarian reserve during chemotherapy	Experimental	In conjunction with chemotherapy	Unknown: small randomized studies and case series report conflicting results Larger randomized trials in progress	$500/month	After Puberty	Does not protect from radiation effects
Donor Embryos	After treatment	Embryos donated by a couple	Standard	Varies; is done in conjunction with IVF	Unknown; higher than that of frozen embryo IVF transfers	$5,000-$7,000 (in addition to costs for IVF)	After Puberty	Available through IVF clinics or private agencies

(continued)

Table 4: Female Options (continued)

Method	Timing	Definition	Medical Status	Time Requirement	Success Rates	Cost	Pubertal Status	Special Considerations
Donor Eggs	After treatment	Eggs donated by a woman	Standard	Varies; is done in conjunction with IVF	40–50%	$5,000–$15,000 (in addition to costs for IVF)	After Puberty	Patient can choose donor based on various characteristics
Gestational Surrogacy	After treatment	Woman carries a pregnancy for another woman or couple	Standard	Varies; time is required to find surrogate and implant embryos	Similar to IVF—approximately 30%	$10,000–$100,000	After Puberty	Legal status varies by state
Adoption	After treatment	Legal proceeding that creates a parent-child relationship	Standard	Varies depending on the type of adoption	Varies greatly	$2,500–$35,000	After Puberty	Can be difficult for cancer survivors given medical history

© Fertile Hope 2007. Reprinted with permission.

Appendix B

Organizations

Cancer and Fertility

Fertile Hope
www.fertilehope.org
P.O. Box 624
New York, NY 10282
(888) 994-HOPE

Infertility

The American Fertility Association
www.theafa.org
305 Madison Avenue, Suite 449
New York, NY 10165
(888) 917-3777

The American Society for Reproductive Medicine
www.asrm.org
1209 Montgomery Highway
Birmingham, AL 35216-2809
(205) 978-5000

The InterNational Council on Infertility Information Dissemination, Inc.
www.inciid.org
P.O. Box 6836
Arlington, VA 22206
(703) 379-9178

The International Premature Ovarian Failure Association
www.pofsupport.org
PO Box 23643
Alexandria, VA 22304
(703) 913-4787

RESOLVE: The National Infertility Association
www.resolve.org
7910 Woodmont Avenue, Suite 1350
Bethesda, MD 20814
(301) 652-8585

Cancer During Pregnancy

Pregnant with Cancer Network
www.pregnantwithcancer.org
PO Box 1243
Buffalo, NY 14220
(800) 743-4471

Web Links

Adoption

The American Academy of Adoption Attorneys
www.adoptionattorneys.org

Child Welfare Information Gateway
www.childwelfare.gov
A comprehensive information service of the Children's Bureau,
Administration for Children and Families, and the U.S.
Department of Health and Human Services.
Click "National Adoption Directory"

National Adoption Information Clearinghouse
http://naic.acf.hhs.gov

Cancer and Fertility

**Association of Online Cancer Resources—Cancer and Fertility
Listserve**
www.acor.org
Type in "fertility" to join the Cancer–Fertility listserve.

ASCO—Recommendations on Fertility Preservation in People Treated for Cancer

www.asco.org

Click "Quality Care & Guidelines" and then "Practice Guidelines" and then "Clinical Practice Guidelines" and then "Survivorship."

ASRM—Patient Fact Sheet on Cancer and Fertility Preservation

www.asrm.org

Click "For Patients" and then "Patient Fact Sheets" and then "Cancer & Fertility Preservation."

Breastcancer.org

http://www.breastcancer.org/fertility_pregnancy_adoption.html

Search "fertility" or see their "Fertility, Pregnancy, Adoption" section.

Fertilitypreservation.org

www.fertilitypreservation.org

LiveStrong—Information on Male and Female Infertility

www.livestrong.org

Search "fertility"

National Cancer Institute Physician Data Query: Sexuality and Reproductive Issues

http://www.cancer.gov/cancertopics/pdq/supportivecare/sexuality

People Living With Cancer

http://www.plwc.org

Search "fertility"

Young Survival Coalition

www.youngsurvival.org

Search "fertility" or log onto their message boards—the fertility sections is one of the most active and robust available today.

Infertility

Fertility Lifelines

www.fertilitylifelines.com

Fertility Neighborhood
www.fertilityneighborhood.com

Fertility Journey
www.fertilityjourney.com

Pediatric Survivors and Infertility

Children's Oncology Group
www.childrensoncologygroup.com
*Click "Long-Term Follow-up Guidelines" and then "Female Health
Issues" or "Male Health Issues."*

Pamphlets and Books

Pamphlets

The following pamphlets are available from Fertile Hope:

Breast Cancer and Fertility
Cancer & Fertility
Cancer & Fertility: A Guide for Young Adults
Cancer & Fertility Resource Guide
Childhood Cancer & Fertility: A Guide for Parents
Gynecologic Cancers & Fertility

Available in Spanish:
La Paternidad y Maternidad Despues del Cancer

Books

Schover, LR. *Sexuality and Fertility After Cancer.* New York: John
Wiley & Sons; 1997.

Glossary

A

Adoption: Process that creates a legal parent–child relationship between persons not related by blood.

Alkylating agents: A family of anti-cancer drugs that interferes with the cell's DNA and inhibits cancer cell growth. This category of chemotherapy medications generally has the worst impact on the reproductive system. Alkylating agents include busulfan, carmustine, carzelesin, cyclophosphamide (also called Cytoxan), ifosfamide, lomustine, melphalan, porfiromycin, and semustine.

Aromatase Inhibitors: Medications that lower the amount of estrogen in the body.

Artificial insemination: Semen is collected and processed in a laboratory and then inserted directly into the woman's cervix or uterus around the time of ovulation to try to achieve pregnancy. This is also called intrauterine insemination (IUI).

Assisted reproductive technologies (ART): A term that covers several high-tech reproductive treatments, including in vitro fertilization.

Azoospermic: The absence of sperm.

B

Bilateral salpingo oophorectomy: Surgery to remove the fallopian tubes plus ovaries.

Biopsy: Removal of a sample of tissue from the body for microscopic examination and diagnosis.

Bone marrow transplant: Procedure in which a patient's bone marrow is destroyed by chemotherapy or radiotherapy and replaced with new bone marrow either from the patient (autologous) or from a matched donor (allogenic).

C

Cerclage: A stitch placed around the cervix, or opening between the uterus and vaginal tract, to keep it closed during pregnancy.

Cervical conization: Surgery to remove a cone-shaped piece of tissue from the cervix and cervical canal. Conization may be used to diagnose or treat a cervical condition. This is also called cone biopsy.

Cervix: The lower section of the uterus that protrudes into the vagina and dilates during labor to allow the passage of the baby.

Conception: Fertilization of a woman's egg by a man's sperm.

Cryobank: A facility where tissues such as sperm, oocytes, and embryos are stored while frozen.

Cryopreservation: The process of storing biological material at low temperatures often for long periods of time. Cryopreservation is often called freezing (e.g., embryo cryopreservation or embryo freezing).

D

Donor eggs: Eggs from the ovaries of a fertile woman that are donated to an infertile woman to be used in an assisted reproductive technology procedure. The donor relinquishes all parental rights to any resulting offspring.

Donor embryos: Embryos donated from one couple to another person or couple. The donors relinquish all parental rights to any offspring.

Donor insemination: Artificial insemination using donor sperm.

Donor sperm: Sperm that is donated by a man who is not a woman's partner for the purpose of producing pregnancy. The donor relinquishes all parental rights to the offspring.

E

Early menopause: Cessation of periods and menopause before the age of 40. Also called *premature ovarian failure* (POF).

Echocardiogram: A noninvasive test in which sound waves are used to produce an image of the heart.

Egg (oocyte): Unfertilized egg that contains the genetic material of the woman.

Egg donation: Eggs from the ovaries of a fertile woman which are donated to an infertile woman to be used in an assisted reproductive technology procedure. The donor relinquishes all parental rights to any resulting offspring. Also called *donor egg.*

Egg freezing: A procedure used to extract mature unfertilized eggs from a woman, freeze them prior to fertilization, and store them for future use.

Egg reserve: A term used to describe the number and quality of eggs in the ovaries. Egg reserve decreases over time until menopause occurs and there are no more viable eggs present. Also called *ovarian reserve.*

Ejaculate: The fluid emitted from a man's penis during orgasm that contains sperm.

Embryo: A fertilized egg from conception through the eighth week of pregnancy.

Embryo donation: Please see *donor embryo.*

Embryo freezing: A procedure used to extract mature, unfertilized eggs from a woman, fertilize the eggs with sperm, and freeze the resulting embryos for future use.

Embryo transfer: The process of placing embryos that have been created and grown in the laboratory into the uterus to try to achieve pregnancy. More than one embryo can be transferred at a time, and thus, the pregnancy rate per transfer is different than the pregnancy rate per embryo or per egg.

Embryologist: A scientist who studies the growth and development of the embryo.

Endometrium: The lining of the uterus which grows and sheds during a normal menstrual cycle and which supports a fetus if a pregnancy occurs.

Estradiol (E2): The principal hormone produced by the growing ovarian follicle. Blood estradiol levels are used to help determine follicle growth during an in vitro fertilization (IVF) cycle.

Estrogen: A hormone produced in both men and women that has a variety of functions. In women, estrogen regulates the development of secondary sex characteristics, including breasts, regulating the monthly cycle of menstruation, and preparing the body for fertilization and reproduction. In breast cancer, estrogen may promote the growth of cancer cells.

F

Fallopian tubes: A pair of tubes attached to the uterus and ovaries, one on each side, where sperm and egg meet in normal conception.

Fertility: The ability to reproduce—in humans, the ability to bear children.

Fertility preservation: Term used to describe procedures that protect a person's fertility or store a person's gametes for future use. These procedures may include egg and embryo freezing,

sperm banking, ovarian transposition, ovarian and testicular tissue freezing, and radical trachelectomy.

Fertility-sparing surgery: General term used to describe specific types of gynecologic surgery for women with ovarian or cervical cancer. For ovarian cancer, this includes removal of only the affected ovary and preservation of the uterus. For cervical cancer, this includes conization and radical trachelectomy.

Fertilization: The penetration of the egg by the sperm and fusion of genetic materials, which results in the development of an embryo.

Fetus: An unborn baby from the eighth week after fertilization until birth.

Follicle: A small sac in the ovary where an egg develops.

Follicle-stimulating hormone (FSH): A hormone produced by the pituitary gland that stimulates the growth of eggs in the ovaries. This hormone is used to help gauge ovarian reserve.

G

Gamete: Male or female reproductive cell—sperm or egg—that contains a haploid set of chromosomes (23).

Gestational surrogacy: An arrangement whereby a woman carries a pregnancy for another person or couple. The *gestational carrier* has the embryo(s) of another couple implanted in her womb. The gestational carrier is not genetically related to the resulting baby. See also *Surrogacy* and *Traditional Surrogacy*.

Gleevec (Imatinib): Medication used to treat chronic myelogenous leukemia (ML), gastrointestinal stromal tumors (GIST), and a number of other malignancies.

GnRH analogues: Hormones secreted by the hypothalamus which controls the pituitary gland's production and release of gonadotropins (hormones involved in reproduction). Synthetic versions of these hormones are sometimes used in assisted reproductive technologies (ART) or to suppress ovarian function in cancer patients.

H

Hematopoietic stem cell transplant (HSCT) : A procedure involving the infusion of either a patient's own stem cells or stem cells from a donor to produce new, healthy marrow. Types of HSCT include bone marrow and stem cell transplants and also umbilical cord blood transplantation. Reproductive damage usually occurs as a result of the high-dose chemotherapy and/or full-body radiation used before infusion of the donor stem cells (see also *bone marrow transplant* and *stem cell transplant*).

Home study: Process where an adoption caseworker interviews potential parents to evaluate whether they are qualified to adopt according to the guidelines of the agency, state, or country where they are adopting from.

Usually background checks, financial reviews, and at least one home visit are part of the process.

Hormone replacement therapy (HRT): The use of synthetic hormones to treat hormone deficiencies. The most common HRT involves estrogen replacement for menopausal women, but testosterone for men can also be used.

Hysterectomy: Surgery to remove the uterus and sometimes the cervix. When the uterus and part or all of the cervix are removed, it is called a total hysterectomy. When only the uterus is removed, it is called a partial hysterectomy.

I

Implantation: The process of attachment of the embryo to the endometrial lining of the uterus.

Impotence: The inability to have an erection of the penis adequate for sexual intercourse. This is also called erectile dysfunction. Being impotent does not mean there is no sperm. Impotence is not the same as infertility, and infertility is not the same as impotence.

Infertility: The inability to conceive after a year of unprotected intercourse or the inability to carry a pregnancy to term.

Insemination: The placement of semen into a woman's uterus, cervix, or vagina to try to achieve pregnancy (see also *artificial insemination* and *intrauterine insemination*).

Intracytoplasmic sperm injection (ICSI): A process in which one sperm is injected into an egg to facilitate fertilization.

Intrauterine insemination (IUI): Process by which semen is collected and then inserted directly into the woman's cervix or uterus to try to achieve pregnancy. This is also called *artificial insemination.*

In vitro fertilization (IVF): A method of assisted reproduction that involves combining an egg with sperm in a laboratory dish. If the egg is fertilized and cell division begins, the resulting embryo is transferred into the woman's uterus.

In vitro maturation (IVM): Process in which immature oocytes (eggs) are obtained from the ovaries and then matured in the laboratory.

M

Menopause: By definition, a woman is menopausal after her periods have stopped for one year. Menopause typically occurs in a woman's late forties to early fifties, but can be accelerated by medical treatments such as chemotherapy and radiation.

Menstrual cycle: The monthly cycle of hormonal changes in the woman during which the uterus is prepared to receive a fertilized egg, the egg is released from an ovary, and blood and tissue are lost via the vagina if a pregnancy does not occur.

Menstruation: Periodic discharge of blood and tissue from the uterus. Until menopause, menstruation occurs approximately every 28 days when a woman is not pregnant.

Miscarriage: Early pregnancy loss, usually before 20-weeks gestation. This is also called *spontaneous abortion.*

Morphology: The physical structure of an organism, including sperm (e.g., shape and size).

Motility: The ability of sperm to move and progress forward through the reproductive tract and fertilize the egg (e.g., speed).

N

Needle aspiration: The use of a thin, hollow needle and syringe to remove body fluid or cells, such as a cell from an embryo, for examination.

O

Obstetrician: A doctor who specializes in pregnancy, labor, and delivery.

Oncologist: A doctor who specializes in the treatment of cancer.

Oocyte: Unfertilized egg that contains the genetic material of the female. A female gametocyte. See also *egg.*

Oophorectomy: Surgery to remove one or both ovaries.

Ovarian failure: The inability of the ovary to respond to hormone stimulation, usually caused by the absence of eggs (oocytes).

Ovarian reserve: A term used to describe the number and quality of eggs in the ovaries. Ovarian reserve decreases over time until menopause occurs and there are no more viable eggs present.

Ovarian shielding: The use of external shields to protect the ovaries from radiation.

Ovarian stimulation: The administration of hormones or fertility medications to mature several eggs in the ovaries.

Ovarian suppression: A treatment to stop the functioning of the ovaries.

Ovarian tissue freezing: A surgical procedure where part or all of an ovary is removed, divided into small strips and frozen for future use to try to restore hormone function and/or achieve pregnancy.

Ovarian transposition: A surgical procedure in which one or both ovaries are moved up into the abdomen so that they are out of the field of radiation.

Ovary (ovaries): The woman's reproductive organ that produces eggs.

Ovulation: The release of a mature egg from its follicle in the ovary. This usually occurs on approximately day 14 of a normal 28-day menstrual cycle.

P

Pituitary gland: A small gland at the base of the brain that secretes hormones and regulates and controls other hormone-secreting glands and many body processes, including growth and reproduction.

Preimplantation genetic diagnosis (PGD): A technique used during IVF to test embryos for genetic disorders before their transfer to the uterus. PGD makes it possible for individuals with serious inherited disorders, including several types of cancer predispositions, to decrease the risk of having a child who is affected by the disorder.

Premature ovarian failure (POF): Cessation of periods and menopause before the age of 40.

Premenstrual syndrome (PMS): Physical and psychological symptoms, including abdominal bloating, breast tenderness, headache, fatigue, irritability, anxiety, and depression, that occur in the days before the onset of menstruation and cease shortly after menses begins.

Prepubescent: At an age before puberty.

Preterm delivery: Birth occurring earlier than 37 weeks of gestation. This is also known as *premature birth*.

Progestin hormonal treatment: Treatment for endometrial cancer to block estrogen, the hormone that endometrial cancer cells need to grow.

Puberty: The process when the development of sexual characteristics occurs and the body becomes capable of reproduction.

R

Radiation shielding: The use of a substance to block or absorb radiation so that tissues behind the shield are protected. Radiation shielding can be used to protect the reproductive system.

Radical trachelectomy: A fertility-sparing surgical procedure used for women with early-stage cervical cancer. The procedure removes most of the cervix but preserves the uterus, allowing the woman to later carry a pregnancy.

Reproductive endocrinologist: A gynecologist who has received board certification in reproductive endocrinology and infertility, following additional fellowship training in the causes, evaluation, and treatment of infertility.

Reproductive system: Organs and tissues involved in the production and maturation of gametes and in their union and subsequent development as offspring. In women, this system includes the ovaries, the fallopian tubes, the uterus, the cervix, and the vagina. The reproductive system in men includes the prostate, the testes, and the penis.

S

Semen: The fluid that is released through the penis during orgasm containing sperm, seminal fluid, and glandular secretions.

Semen analysis: The microscopic examination of semen to determine the number of sperm (sperm count), their shape (morphology), and their ability to move (motility).

Shared risk program: Payment option for people when their insurance does not cover in vitro fertilization (IVF). The patient pays a fixed up-front cost for a set number of IVF attempts. If there is no successful pregnancy after the IVF attempts, the money is refunded.

Slow freezing: A technique used to freeze eggs and embryos. Cooling and warming rates are controlled to reduce the risk of ice crystal formation and damage to the egg or embryo.

Sperm: A man's reproductive cells, also called gametes.

Sperm banking: Freezing sperm for use in the future. This procedure can allow men to father children after loss of fertility.

Sperm count: A basic assessment of sperm function, primarily involving counting the number of sperm, as well as its motility and morphology.

Stem cells: Undifferentiated, immature cells that develop into specialized cells.

Stem cell transplant: A procedure involving the infusion of either a patient's own stem cells or stem cells from a donor to produce new, healthy marrow. Stem cell transplantation usually refers to a procedure which involves collection of the stem cells from the blood stream; if stem cells are harvested from the bone marrow, the procedure is referred to as a bone marrow transplant.

Sterile: Unable to produce children.

Surrogate: A woman who carries a pregnancy for another person or couple. A surrogate can either be inseminated with the sperm of a man who is not her partner in order to conceive and carry his (and his partner's) child (traditional surrogacy), or she can have the embryo(s) of another couple implanted in her uterus (gestation surrogacy) and carry the pregnancy for the couple (see also *traditional surrogacy* and *gestational surrogacy*).

T

Tamoxifen: A medication that blocks the effects of estrogen on many organs, such as the breast. Tamoxifen can be used with standard fertility medications to block the effects of estrogen.

Testicles: A man's sex glands located in the scrotum, which produce sperm and testosterone.

Testicular biopsy: A surgical procedure that allows for microscopic examination of testicular tissue. The tissue, removed through a small incision in the scrotum, can often identify sperm and/or help determine the causes of infertility and suggest a course of treatment.

Testicular sperm extraction (TESE): A procedure for obtaining sperm by removing a small piece of testicular tissue through a small cut in the scrotum or by retrieving sperm directly from the testes.

Testicular tissue freezing: A surgical procedure to remove testicular tissue from the testes and freeze it for future use.

Testosterone: A hormone that promotes the development and maintenance of men's sex characteristics.

Traditional surrogacy: Arrangement whereby a woman is inseminated with the sperm of a man who is not her partner in order to conceive and carry his (and his partner's) child. Through this procedure, the surrogate is genetically and legally related to the baby; her parental rights must be surrendered in order for the partner of the biological father to be recognized as a legal parent.

U

Ultrasound: Procedure in which high-energy sound waves are bounced off internal tissues or organs and make echoes. The echo patterns are shown on the screen of an ultrasound machine, forming a picture of body tissues called a sonogram.

Uterus: The small, hollow, pear-shaped organ in a woman's pelvis. This is the organ in which a fetus develops. It is also called a *womb*.

V

Vitrification: Method of egg freezing that involves rapid cooling with high concentrations of cryoprotectants to reduce the formation of ice crystals. Also called fast freezing.

INDEX

Index

Index